I0775212

ESSENTIAL PLANT-POWERED PROTEIN

Dietary Guidelines for All Ages and Nutritional Fundamentals

By

Calvin M. Duncan

All rights reserved. No part of this publication may be reproduced, distributed, or transmitted in any form or by any means, including photocopying, recording or other electronic or mechanical methods, without the prior written permission of the publisher, except in the case of brief quotation embodied in critical reviews and certain other noncommercial uses permitted by copyright law

Copyright by Calvin M. Duncan 2023

Table Of Contents

Introduction
The Rise of Plant-Powered Nutrition

In recent years, there has been a notable shift in dietary patterns as more individuals embrace plant-powered nutrition. This dietary approach places a strong emphasis on incorporating plant-based foods as the foundation of one's daily meals, steering away from traditional diets centered around animal products. The motivations behind this shift are diverse, ranging from health concerns and ethical considerations to environmental sustainability. This essay explores the multifaceted rise of plant-powered nutrition, delving into the health benefits, ethical dimensions, and environmental implications that have propelled this dietary movement into the mainstream.

One of the primary drivers behind the surge in plant-powered nutrition is the growing awareness of its numerous health benefits. Research consistently indicates that a plant-centric diet can contribute to overall well-being and reduce the risk of various chronic diseases. Fruits, vegetables, legumes, nuts, and seeds offer a rich array of essential vitamins, minerals, fiber, and antioxidants that play a crucial role in maintaining optimal health.

Plant-based diets have been associated with lower rates of cardiovascular diseases, hypertension, and Type 2 diabetes. The abundant fiber in plant foods not only promotes digestive health but also helps in weight management by inducing a feeling of satiety. Moreover, the phytochemicals present in plant-based foods have been linked to anti-inflammatory and anti-cancer properties, further underlining the potential of plant-powered nutrition in disease prevention and management.

Beyond personal health, many individuals are drawn to plant-powered nutrition due to ethical considerations related to animal welfare. The conventional methods of factory farming and industrial animal agriculture have come under scrutiny for their environmental impact and the ethical treatment of animals. As awareness of these issues grows, more people are choosing plant-based diets as a way to align their food choices with ethical principles.

The ethical dimensions of plant-powered nutrition extend beyond the treatment of animals to include broader concerns about sustainable and humane practices. Plant-based diets, which rely on a variety of crops and plant sources, have a lower environmental footprint compared to the resource-intensive nature of animal agriculture. This aligns with the ethical imperative of minimizing one's ecological impact and promoting a more sustainable food system.

The environmental impact of dietary choices has become a central focus in discussions about sustainable living. Plant-powered nutrition stands out as a key solution in addressing environmental concerns associated with traditional diets heavy in animal products. Livestock farming, particularly cattle rearing, contributes significantly to deforestation, greenhouse gas emissions, and water pollution.

By choosing plant-based alternatives, individuals can play a role in mitigating the environmental consequences of food production. Plant-powered diets generally have a lower carbon footprint, require less land and water, and contribute less to deforestation. This shift towards plant-centric eating aligns with global efforts to combat climate change and promotes a more sustainable and environmentally friendly approach to food consumption.

While the rise of plant-powered nutrition is gaining momentum, it is not without its challenges and misconceptions. One common misconception is the belief that plant-based diets lack essential nutrients, particularly protein. However, with careful planning and a varied selection of plant foods, individuals can meet their nutritional needs and obtain an adequate protein intake from plant sources such as legumes, tofu, tempeh, and plant-based protein supplements.

Another challenge involves the accessibility and affordability of plant-based options, as some communities may have limited access to fresh produce or plant-based alternatives. Addressing these challenges requires a concerted effort from policymakers, communities, and the food industry to make plant-powered nutrition more accessible and inclusive.

As the popularity of plant-powered nutrition grows, innovation in the food industry has played a pivotal role in expanding the variety and accessibility of plant-based options. Plant-based alternatives to traditional animal products, such as plant-based meats, dairy substitutes, and egg alternatives, have proliferated in the market. These innovations not only cater to those transitioning to a plant-based diet but also appeal to a broader audience, including flexitarians seeking to reduce their meat consumption.

Advancements in food technology and culinary creativity have led to the development of plant-based products that closely mimic the taste, texture, and nutritional profile of their animal-derived counterparts. This not only makes plant-powered nutrition more appealing but also addresses concerns about sacrificing taste and convenience when adopting a plant-based lifestyle.

One of the misconceptions about plant-powered nutrition is that it involves a limited and monotonous range of foods. In reality, plant-based diets offer a diverse and exciting array of culinary possibilities. The richness of fruits, vegetables, whole grains, legumes, nuts, and seeds allows for a broad spectrum of flavors, textures, and cuisines.

Exploring plant-powered nutrition encourages individuals to rediscover traditional and international dishes, experiment with new ingredients, and cultivate a deeper appreciation for the natural flavors inherent in plant-based foods. The culinary diversity of plant-powered diets challenges preconceived notions about restrictive eating and showcases the abundance of delicious options available to those who choose to embrace a plant-centric lifestyle.

The rise of plant-powered nutrition is not merely a dietary trend but also a reflection of broader cultural and social shifts in attitudes toward food. Social media, documentaries, and influential figures promoting plant-based living have contributed to the dissemination of information and the creation of a supportive community for those exploring or adopting plant-powered diets.

Cultural norms around food are evolving as plant-based options become more mainstream and accessible. Restaurants, cafes, and food establishments increasingly offer diverse plant-based

menu items, accommodating the growing demand for alternatives to traditional animal-based dishes. This cultural shift signifies a changing relationship with food, emphasizing sustainability, health consciousness, and ethical considerations in dietary choices.

The rise of plant-powered nutrition represents a multifaceted movement driven by considerations of health, ethics, and the environment. As individuals increasingly recognize the health benefits of plant-based diets, the ethical dimensions of food choices, and the environmental impact of traditional agricultural practices, plant-powered nutrition has emerged as a holistic and sustainable approach to eating.

The journey toward plant-powered nutrition involves addressing challenges, dispelling misconceptions, and fostering innovation in the food industry. Culinary diversity, coupled with cultural and social shifts, is reshaping the way we think about food and challenging the notion that a plant-based diet is limiting or exclusive.

In embracing plant-powered nutrition, individuals contribute not only to their own well-being but also to a more sustainable and compassionate global food system. As the movement continues to gain momentum, it holds the potential to transform our relationship with food, redefine culinary traditions, and pave the way toward a healthier, more ethical, and environmentally conscious future.

The Significance of Dietary Guidelines for All Ages

Dietary guidelines play a pivotal role in shaping the nutritional habits and health outcomes of individuals across the lifespan. As our understanding of nutrition evolves, so too do the recommendations that guide dietary choices. These guidelines are essential tools for promoting optimal health, preventing chronic diseases, and addressing the specific nutritional needs of different age groups. This essay explores the significance of dietary guidelines for all ages, examining how these recommendations contribute to overall well-being and establish the foundation for a healthy life.

Dietary guidelines serve as evidence-based recommendations developed by health professionals and nutrition experts to guide individuals in making informed food choices. These guidelines are designed to address the nutritional requirements of diverse populations and are typically issued by

government health agencies, such as the U.S. Department of Agriculture (USDA) or the World Health Organization (WHO). The foundational principles of dietary guidelines encompass a balanced intake of macronutrients (carbohydrates, proteins, and fats), micronutrients (vitamins and minerals), and other essential components such as fiber and water.

The significance of these guidelines lies in their ability to provide a framework for individuals to meet their nutritional needs, support growth and development, and reduce the risk of diet-related diseases. By offering scientifically informed recommendations, dietary guidelines empower individuals to make choices that align with their health goals, regardless of age or life stage.

Dietary guidelines tailored to children and adolescents are of paramount importance in establishing lifelong health habits. Early nutrition plays a crucial role in growth, cognitive development, and the prevention of childhood obesity and related health issues. Guidelines for this age group typically emphasize the importance of a well-balanced diet that includes a variety of fruits, vegetables, whole grains, lean proteins, and dairy or dairy alternatives.

Furthermore, childhood dietary guidelines often provide specific recommendations for key nutrients, such as calcium and vitamin D, which are essential for bone development, and iron, critical for cognitive function. Establishing healthy eating patterns during childhood not only supports immediate well-being but also lays the groundwork for lifelong habits that can prevent diet-related diseases in adulthood.

As individuals transition from childhood to adolescence, their nutritional needs undergo significant changes. Dietary guidelines for adolescents recognize the increased demands for energy, protein, and other nutrients associated with the growth spurt and puberty. Adolescents are encouraged to make nutrient-dense food choices that provide essential vitamins and minerals while being mindful of energy balance to prevent excessive weight gain.

Additionally, dietary guidelines for this age group often address the growing concern of inadequate intake of fruits, vegetables, and whole grains. Encouraging healthy eating patterns during adolescence not only supports physical development but also fosters cognitive function and establishes habits that can influence long-term health outcomes.

The significance of dietary guidelines persists into adulthood, where they play a crucial role in preventing chronic diseases and promoting overall well-being. Adult dietary guidelines focus on achieving and maintaining a healthy body weight, reducing the risk of cardiovascular diseases, managing blood pressure, and preventing nutrient deficiencies associated with aging.

For adults, dietary guidelines often include recommendations on portion sizes, moderation of added sugars and saturated fats, and increased consumption of nutrient-dense foods. The emphasis on maintaining a diverse and balanced diet becomes even more critical as individuals navigate the challenges of busy lifestyles, work-related stress, and changes in metabolic rate that come with aging.

The significance of dietary guidelines extends to the unique nutritional needs of pregnant and lactating individuals. Proper nutrition during these critical periods not only supports the health of the mother but also contributes to the optimal development of the fetus and the well-being of the

newborn. Guidelines for pregnancy highlight the increased need for certain nutrients such as folic acid, iron, and calcium, while lactation guidelines focus on sustaining maternal health and providing essential nutrients through breast milk.

Nutritional adequacy during pregnancy and lactation is crucial for preventing birth defects, supporting fetal growth and development, and ensuring the health of both mother and child. Dietary guidelines provide expectant and nursing mothers with valuable information to make informed choices that support the unique demands of these life stages.

As individuals age, their nutritional needs and dietary challenges evolve, making dietary guidelines for older adults particularly significant. Guidelines for this demographic address factors such as decreased muscle mass, changes in metabolism, and the increased risk of chronic diseases. Adequate protein intake, along with calcium and vitamin D, becomes a focal point to support bone health and muscle mass.

Moreover, dietary guidelines for older adults often stress the importance of hydration, fiber intake to support digestive health, and the role of antioxidants in mitigating age-related oxidative stress. By addressing the specific nutritional needs of older individuals, dietary guidelines contribute to healthy aging, disease prevention, and the maintenance of a high quality of life.

Dietary guidelines play a pivotal role in the prevention and management of chronic diseases, such as cardiovascular diseases, diabetes, and certain cancers. Recommendations often center around reducing the intake of saturated and trans fats, sodium, and added sugars while promoting the consumption of fruits, vegetables, whole grains, and lean proteins. These guidelines empower individuals to make dietary choices that can positively impact their health outcomes and reduce the risk of developing debilitating conditions.

For individuals with existing health conditions, dietary guidelines offer tailored recommendations to manage their conditions through nutrition. For example, individuals with diabetes may receive guidance on carbohydrate intake and blood sugar management, while those with hypertension may be advised to follow a low-sodium diet. The significance of these guidelines in disease management is evident in their ability to complement medical interventions and improve overall health outcomes.

Dietary guidelines recognize the diverse cultural backgrounds and dietary practices of populations worldwide. The significance of these guidelines lies in their adaptability to different cultural contexts, ensuring that recommendations are both culturally sensitive and relevant to diverse communities. By acknowledging the variety of foods and culinary traditions, dietary guidelines foster dietary diversity and inclusivity.

Cultural sensitivity in dietary guidelines extends beyond individual choices to community-level considerations. Recognizing the role of cultural practices in shaping dietary habits allows for the development of guidelines that respect traditions while promoting nutritional well-being. This cultural inclusivity enhances the effectiveness and acceptance of dietary recommendations across diverse populations.

It serve as a critical educational tool, contributing to the promotion of nutrition literacy at both individual and community levels. Understanding the principles of a balanced diet, the importance of specific nutrients, and the relationship between diet and health empowers individuals to make informed choices about their food intake.

Nutrition education based on dietary guidelines is particularly valuable in schools, healthcare settings, and community programs. By disseminating accurate and accessible information, these guidelines foster a culture of health-conscious decision-making, empowering individuals to take control of their nutritional well-being. Nutrition literacy, in turn, has the potential to reduce the prevalence of diet-related diseases and improve overall public health.

The significance of dietary guidelines extends beyond individual health to influence public health policy and planning. Government agencies use these guidelines as a foundation for developing nutrition policies, school meal programs, and public health initiatives. By aligning policy decisions with evidence-based dietary recommendations, governments can address public health challenges and promote the well-being of entire populations.

Furthermore, dietary guidelines contribute to the development of nutrition standards in food labeling and advertising. Clear and informative labeling helps consumers make healthier choices when purchasing food pproduct, contributing to the prevention of diet-related diseases. The integration of dietary guidelines into public health policy reflects a commitment to creating environments that support healthy food choices and lifestyles.

The significance of dietary guidelines for all ages cannot be overstated, as they serve as a cornerstone for promoting health, preventing disease, and fostering nutrition literacy. From childhood through the various life stages to older adulthood, dietary guidelines provide valuable insights into the nutritional requirements specific to each age group. By addressing the diverse needs of individuals across the lifespan, these guidelines contribute to the development of lifelong healthy habits and the prevention of diet-related diseases.

The adaptability of dietary guidelines to diverse cultural contexts ensures that they are inclusive and relevant to populations worldwide. Additionally, their role in disease prevention and management, coupled with their influence on public health policy, highlights their far-reaching impact on the overall well-being of communities.

In an era where the global burden of diet-related diseases is on the rise, the significance of evidence-based dietary guidelines cannot be overstated. As our understanding of nutrition continues to evolve, so too will the guidelines that guide us toward healthier, more sustainable, and fulfilling lives. Embracing the principles of dietary guidelines is not merely a personal choice but a collective commitment to a healthier and more resilient society.

Chapter One
Understanding Proteins and Plant-Based Proteins

Proteins are fundamental to the very fabric of life, serving as intricate molecular machines that play crucial roles in the structure, function, and regulation of cells and tissues. Composed of amino acids, proteins are essential macromolecules that contribute to the maintenance and vitality of living organisms. This essay explores the nature of proteins, delving into their diverse functions and the significance they hold in the context of human nutrition. Additionally, the focus shifts to plant-based proteins, exploring their sources, nutritional value, and the growing interest in incorporating them into a balanced diet.

Understanding Proteins

Proteins are large, complex molecules composed of amino acids, often referred to as the building blocks of proteins. There are 20 different amino acids that can combine in various sequences to form a vast array of proteins, each with its unique structure and function. The sequence of amino acids determines the three-dimensional structure of a protein, which, in turn, dictates its specific role in biological processes.

Functions of Proteins

The functions of proteins are incredibly diverse, reflecting their critical roles in nearly every biological process. Some of the key functions include:

1. Structural Support: Proteins provide structural support to cells and tissues. Collagen, for example, is a fibrous protein that forms the structural framework of connective tissues in the body, such as skin, tendons, and bones.

2. Enzymatic Activity: Many proteins function as enzymes, facilitating and accelerating biochemical reactions in the body. Enzymes are involved in processes such as digestion, energy production, and DNA replication.

3. Transportation: Proteins play a vital role in transporting molecules across cell membranes. Hemoglobin, a protein in red blood cells, transports oxygen from the lungs to tissues throughout the body.

4. Immune Defense: Antibodies, a type of protein, are crucial components of the immune system. They recognize and neutralize foreign substances, such as bacteria and viruses, helping the body defend against infections.

5. Cell Signaling: Proteins are involved in cell signaling, transmitting signals within and between cells. Hormones, which regulate various physiological processes, are often proteins.

6. Muscle Contraction: Proteins, particularly actin and myosin, are essential for muscle contraction. This function is vital for movement and locomotion.

Nutritional Importance of Proteins

In addition to their diverse biological functions, proteins are integral to human nutrition. Proteins serve as a source of essential amino acids, which the body cannot produce on its own and must obtain through the diet. Amino acids are classified into essential and non-essential categories, with essential amino acids being crucial for the synthesis of proteins that the body cannot synthesize independently.

Dietary proteins are derived from both animal and plant sources. Animal proteins, found in meat, dairy, and eggs, are considered complete proteins as they contain all essential amino acids in sufficient quantities. Plant proteins, on the other hand, may lack one or more essential amino acids, making it important for individuals following plant-based diets to ensure a varied and balanced intake of protein sources.

Plant-Based Proteins

As interest in plant-based diets continues to grow for reasons ranging from health and ethical concerns to environmental sustainability, the spotlight on plant-based proteins has intensified. Plant-based proteins are derived from a variety of plant sources, offering a wealth of options for individuals seeking to incorporate more plant-based foods into their diets.

Sources of Plant-Based Proteins

1. Legumes: Beans, lentils, chickpeas, and peas are rich sources of plant-based proteins. They are not only high in protein but also provide fiber, vitamins, and minerals.

2. Nuts and Seeds: Almonds, peanuts, chia seeds, flaxseeds, and pumpkin seeds are examples of plant-based protein sources that also offer healthy fats, fiber, and micronutrients.

3. Whole Grains: Quinoa, brown rice, oats, and barley are whole grains that contribute to protein intake while providing complex carbohydrates for sustained energy.

4. Soy Products: Tofu, tempeh, and edamame are derived from soybeans and are versatile plant-based protein sources. They are complete proteins, containing all essential amino acids.

5. Vegetables: Some vegetables, such as spinach, broccoli, and Brussels sprouts, contain notable amounts of protein in addition to other essential nutrients.

Nutritional Value of Plant-Based Proteins

Plant-based proteins offer numerous health benefits due to their unique nutritional profiles. While they may not always provide complete proteins, combining different plant-based protein sources over the course of the day can ensure a well-rounded amino acid intake. Additionally, plant-based proteins often come packaged with other beneficial nutrients such as fiber, antioxidants, and phytochemicals.

1. Heart Health: Many plant-based proteins, such as those found in legumes and nuts, have been associated with lower risks of heart disease. Their fiber content, coupled with healthy fats, contributes to cardiovascular health.

2. Weight Management: Plant-based proteins can be beneficial for weight management due to their lower calorie and saturated fat content compared to some animal-based proteins. The fiber in plant-based foods also promotes feelings of fullness.

3. Digestive Health: The fiber in plant-based foods supports digestive health by promoting regular bowel movements and fostering a healthy gut microbiome.

4. Reduced Environmental Impact: Choosing plant-based proteins can contribute to environmental sustainability by reducing the environmental footprint associated with animal agriculture.

Challenges and Considerations

While plant-based proteins offer numerous health benefits, there are challenges and considerations associated with exclusively relying on plant sources for protein. One key consideration is the amino acid profile, as certain plant sources may lack one or more essential amino acids. However, this challenge can be mitigated by consuming a variety of plant-based foods to ensure a balanced intake of amino acids.

Another consideration is the bioavailability of nutrients. Some plant compounds, such as phytates and oxalates, can limit the absorption of certain minerals like iron and calcium. However, thoughtful food choices and dietary planning can help address these considerations and ensure optimal nutrient absorption.

Conclusion

In conclusion, proteins stand as the essential building blocks of life, contributing to the structure, function, and regulation of biological processes. The significance of proteins in human nutrition is undeniable, with their diverse functions supporting overall health and well-being. Plant-based proteins, derived from sources such as legumes, nuts, seeds, soy, and vegetables, offer a sustainable and healthful alternative to animal-based proteins.

The nutritional value of plant-based proteins extends beyond their protein content, as they come bundled with fiber, vitamins, minerals, and other beneficial compounds. As the interest in plant-based diets continues to rise, understanding the nutritional importance of both animal and plant-based proteins becomes crucial for making informed dietary choices. Whether one chooses to follow a plant-based diet or include a mix of plant and animal proteins, the key lies in embracing a diverse and balanced approach to nutrition that meets individual health goals and supports overall well-being.

Chapter Two

Amino Acids: The Building Blocks of Proteins

Amino acids stand as the fundamental constituents of proteins, playing a pivotal role in the structure, function, and regulation of biological processes. As the building blocks of life, these molecules are essential for the existence and vitality of living organisms. This essay explores the intricate world of amino acids, delving into their classification, structural characteristics, and the crucial role they play in the formation of proteins. Additionally, we will explore the significance of amino acids in human nutrition, the genetic code that governs their synthesis, and the broader implications for health and well-being.

Classification of Amino Acids

Amino acids are organic compounds characterized by the presence of both an amino group (-NH2) and a carboxyl group (-COOH). The central carbon atom, known as the alpha carbon, is also bonded to a hydrogen atom and a side chain, denoted as the "R" group. It is the nature of this side chain that distinguishes one amino acid from another, imparting unique characteristics to each.

Amino acids can be classified based on the properties of their side chains, leading to several categories:

1. Non-Polar Amino Acids: These amino acids have hydrophobic side chains and are insoluble in water. Examples include glycine, alanine, valine, leucine, and isoleucine.

2. Polar Amino Acids: Amino acids with polar but uncharged side chains are hydrophilic and can form hydrogen bonds with water molecules. Serine, threonine, and asparagine are examples of polar amino acids.

3. Negatively Charged (Acidic) Amino Acids: Amino acids with acidic side chains carry a negative charge. Examples include aspartic acid and glutamic acid.

4. Positively Charged (Basic) Amino Acids: Amino acids with basic side chains are positively charged. Lysine, arginine, and histidine fall into this category.

The diversity in the side chain structures contributes to the unique properties and functions of each amino acid within the context of protein synthesis and biological activities.

The Peptide Bond: Linking Amino Acids in Proteins

The linkage of amino acids is a critical step in the formation of proteins. Amino acids are connected through peptide bonds, which form between the carboxyl group of one amino acid and the amino group of another. This condensation reaction results in the release of a water molecule.

The resulting structure, known as a dipeptide, consists of two amino acids joined by a peptide bond. As additional amino acids are added through peptide bond formation, a polypeptide chain is formed. Polypeptides can range in length from a few amino acids to thousands, ultimately folding into a specific three-dimensional structure that defines the protein's function.

Proteins: The Three-Dimensional Conformation

The sequence of amino acids in a polypeptide chain determines its primary structure. However, the primary structure is just the beginning of a protein's journey toward functionality. Proteins undergo intricate folding to attain specific three-dimensional structures, which are critical for their biological activity.

The folding process involves interactions between amino acids, driven by forces such as hydrogen bonding, van der Waals forces, ionic interactions, and hydrophobic interactions. These interactions result in the formation of secondary structures, including alpha helices and beta sheets, which further fold into the protein's tertiary structure.

The quaternary structure of proteins refers to the arrangement of multiple polypeptide chains (subunits) in a multi-subunit complex. Not all proteins have quaternary structures; some consist of a single polypeptide chain (monomer), while others require the interaction of multiple chains to achieve their functional form.

The significance of the three-dimensional conformation lies in its direct influence on a protein's function. Proteins are highly specific in their interactions, and their ability to recognize and bind to other molecules, such as substrates or signaling molecules, is intricately tied to their unique shapes.

Genetic Code: A Blueprint for Amino Acid Sequences

The sequence of amino acids in a protein is dictated by the information encoded in the genetic material. In living organisms, DNA serves as the repository of genetic information, and the genetic code governs the translation of this information into the synthesis of proteins.

The genetic code is a set of rules that relates the sequence of nucleotide triplets (codons) in DNA to the sequence of amino acids in a protein. Each codon corresponds to a specific amino acid or signals the start or end of protein synthesis. There are 64 possible codons, and each codon codes for one of the 20 amino acids or serves as a start or stop signal.

The specificity of the genetic code ensures the accurate and precise synthesis of proteins based on the instructions encoded in the DNA. The process of transcription involves the synthesis of messenger RNA (mRNA) from a DNA template, and translation translates the mRNA sequence into a sequence of amino acids during protein synthesis.

Human Nutrition and Amino Acids

Amino acids play a vital role in human nutrition as they are essential components of the proteins that contribute to the structure and function of the body. While the body can synthesize some amino acids, others must be obtained through the diet and are termed essential amino acids.

Essential amino acids include:

1. Histidine

2. Isoleucine

3. Leucine

4. Lysine

5. Methionine

6. Phenylalanine

7. Threonine

8. Tryptophan

9. Valine

These essential amino acids must be sourced from dietary proteins, highlighting the importance of a well-balanced and diverse diet for meeting nutritional needs.

Complete Proteins vs. Incomplete Proteins

Dietary proteins are derived from both animal and plant sources. Animal proteins, found in meat, dairy, and eggs, are considered complete proteins as they contain all essential amino acids in sufficient quantities. These proteins are particularly valuable for individuals who rely on animal products as primary protein sources.

Plant proteins, on the other hand, may lack one or more essential amino acids, making them incomplete proteins. Common plant-based protein sources include legumes, grains, nuts, and seeds. While individual plant foods may be deficient in certain essential amino acids, combining different plant-based protein sources over the course of the day can ensure a balanced intake of all essential amino acids.

Protein Complementation: Achieving Amino Acid Balance

Protein complementation is a dietary strategy that involves combining different plant-based protein sources to ensure a more balanced intake of essential amino acids. By pairing foods that have complementary amino acid profiles, individuals following plant-based diets can create a more nutritionally complete protein source.

For example, combining legumes (such as beans or lentils) with grains (such as rice or wheat) can provide a more balanced amino acid profile. Legumes are rich in lysine but lower in methionine, while grains have the opposite profile. Together, they complement each other, resulting in a more nutritionally complete protein source.

This approach highlights the importance of dietary planning for individuals who choose plant-based or vegetarian diets, ensuring they receive an adequate and balanced intake of essential amino acids.

Health Implications of Amino Acids

Amino acids play a crucial role in maintaining health, and their availability influences various physiological processes. Some notable health implications of amino acids include:

1. Muscle Synthesis and Repair: Amino acids are essential for the synthesis and repair of muscle tissue. This is particularly relevant in the context of physical activity, exercise, and the recovery process following muscle damage.

2. Enzyme Function: Many enzymes, which are proteins that facilitate biochemical reactions, rely on specific amino acid sequences for their catalytic activity. Amino acids contribute to the functionality of enzymes involved in digestion, energy production, and other metabolic processes.

3. Immune System Function: Amino acids are integral to the function of antibodies, immune cells, and other components of the immune system. Adequate protein intake is crucial for supporting immune responses and defense against infections.

4. Neurotransmitter Synthesis: Certain amino acids serve as precursors for the synthesis of neurotransmitters, which are essential for proper nervous system function. For example, tryptophan is a precursor for serotonin, a neurotransmitter involved in mood regulation.

5.*Hormone Production: Amino acids contribute to the synthesis of hormones that regulate various physiological processes, including growth, metabolism, and stress responses. For instance, tyrosine is a precursor for thyroid hormones.

6. Blood Sugar Regulation: Amino acids, particularly branched-chain amino acids (BCAAs), play a role in regulating blood sugar levels. They can be used as an energy source during periods of increased energy demand or fasting.

7. Wound Healing: Amino acids are essential for the synthesis of collagen and other proteins involved in tissue repair and wound healing. Adequate protein intake supports the body's ability to recover from injuries.

Imbalances in amino acid intake can have implications for health. Deficiencies in essential amino acids, whether due to inadequate dietary intake or impaired absorption, can lead to a range of health issues, including compromised immune function, muscle wasting, and impaired growth in children.

On the other hand, excessive intake of certain amino acids, often associated with the overconsumption of protein supplements or specific dietary patterns, may have adverse effects. High intake of certain amino acids, such as methionine, has been linked to potential health risks, including cardiovascular issues.

Amino Acids in Disease and Therapeutics

The role of amino acids extends beyond basic physiological functions to influence various disease processes. Imbalances in amino acid metabolism have been implicated in the development of certain diseases, and targeted interventions involving amino acid supplementation or restriction are explored in therapeutic contexts.

1. Inborn Errors of Metabolism: Genetic mutations affecting enzymes involved in amino acid metabolism can lead to inborn errors of metabolism. Conditions such as phenylketonuria (PKU) result in the inability to metabolize phenylalanine, leading to its accumulation and potential neurological damage. Early detection and dietary management, often involving restriction of specific amino acids, are crucial for managing these conditions.

2. Neurological Disorders: Amino acid imbalances have been implicated in various neurological disorders. For example, abnormalities in the metabolism of neurotransmitter-related amino acids like glutamate and gamma-aminobutyric acid (GABA) are associated with conditions such as epilepsy and certain neurodegenerative diseases.

3. Cancer: Amino acid metabolism is altered in cancer cells, and specific amino acids, such as glutamine, play a role in supporting the rapid proliferation of cancer cells. Targeting amino acid metabolism is an area of interest in cancer research for potential therapeutic interventions.

4. Cardiovascular Disease: Elevated levels of certain amino acids, such as homocysteine, have been linked to an increased risk of cardiovascular disease. Amino acid-related pathways are

explored in the context of cardiovascular health, and interventions aimed at modulating these pathways are under investigation.

5. Metabolic Syndrome and Diabetes: Amino acids, particularly BCAAs, have been implicated in metabolic syndrome and insulin resistance. Imbalances in amino acid metabolism are associated with the development of type 2 diabetes and related metabolic disorders.

These connections between amino acids and various diseases highlight the intricate relationships within the body's biochemical pathways. Targeting specific amino acid-related pathways is an area of ongoing research, with the potential for developing novel therapeutic strategies for a range of health conditions.

In summary, amino acids serve as the indispensable building blocks of proteins, contributing to the structure and function of living organisms. The classification of amino acids based on their side chain properties reflects their diverse roles in biological processes. The peptide bond, formed through condensation reactions between amino acids, connects them into polypeptide chains that fold into complex three-dimensional structures.

The genetic code provides the blueprint for the sequence of amino acids in proteins, ensuring the accurate translation of genetic information into functional molecules. Amino acids are crucial in human nutrition, with essential amino acids requiring dietary intake to meet nutritional needs. The distinction between complete and incomplete proteins emphasizes the importance of dietary planning, particularly in the context of plant-based diets.

Beyond their foundational role in protein synthesis, amino acids influence various physiological processes with implications for health and disease. The interplay between amino acids and disease pathways is an active area of research, offering insights into potential therapeutic interventions for a range of conditions.

As our understanding of amino acids continues to deepen, their significance in the intricate web of molecular interactions within the body becomes increasingly apparent. From the intricate folds of proteins to the delicate balance in metabolic pathways, amino acids stand as molecular architects, shaping the foundation of life itself.

Chapter Three

Plant-Based Protein Breakfast Ideas

Breakfast, often hailed as the most important meal of the day, sets the tone for our energy levels, metabolism, and overall well-being. For individuals following a plant-based diet, ensuring an adequate intake of protein is essential for a balanced and nourishing start to the day. This essay explores a diverse array of plant-based protein breakfast ideas, highlighting the rich variety of options available for those seeking to embrace a plant-powered morning routine. From traditional favorites to innovative and globally inspired dishes, these breakfast ideas showcase the versatility and nutritional benefits of plant-based proteins.

The Importance of Plant-Based Proteins in Breakfast

Plant-based proteins play a crucial role in supporting overall health and meeting the nutritional needs of individuals who follow vegetarian, vegan, or plant-centric diets. Unlike animal proteins, which are complete proteins containing all essential amino acids, some plant proteins may lack certain amino acids. Therefore, it's important for individuals relying on plant-based sources to include a variety of protein-rich foods throughout the day to ensure a well-rounded amino acid profile.

Breakfast is an opportune time to incorporate plant-based proteins, as it kickstarts the day with sustained energy and provides the body with the necessary nutrients for optimal functioning. Plant-based proteins offer additional benefits, such as being rich in fiber, antioxidants, vitamins, and minerals, contributing to a well-balanced and nutrient-dense breakfast.

Plant-Based Protein Sources for Breakfast

Before exploring specific breakfast ideas, it's helpful to understand the diverse plant-based protein sources available:

1. Legumes: Beans, lentils, chickpeas, and peas are excellent sources of plant-based proteins. They can be incorporated into various breakfast dishes, providing a hearty and satisfying protein boost.

2. Tofu and Tempeh: Tofu and tempeh, both derived from soybeans, are versatile plant-based proteins that can be used in savory and sweet breakfast recipes. They absorb flavors well and can be prepared in a variety of ways.

3. Nuts and Seeds: Almonds, walnuts, chia seeds, flaxseeds, hemp seeds, and pumpkin seeds are nutrient-dense options rich in protein, healthy fats, and essential nutrients.

4. Whole Grains: Quinoa, oats, brown rice, and farro are whole grains that not only provide complex carbohydrates but also contribute to the protein content of breakfast dishes.

5. Plant-Based Yogurts: Yogurts made from almond, soy, coconut, or oat milk are good sources of plant-based protein. They can be enjoyed on their own or used as a base for various breakfast creations.

6. Plant-Based Milk: Almond, soy, oat, and pea milk are examples of plant-based milk alternatives that can be used in place of dairy milk, offering protein along with other essential nutrients.

7. Vegetables: Certain vegetables, such as spinach, broccoli, and mushrooms, contain notable amounts of protein and can be incorporated into breakfast recipes for added nutrition.

Plant-Based Protein Breakfast Ideas

1. Classic Overnight Oats with Almond Butter and Berries:

   - Ingredients: Rolled oats, almond milk, chia seeds, almond butter, fresh berries.

   - Method: Combine oats, almond milk, and chia seeds in a jar. Refrigerate overnight. In the morning, top with almond butter and fresh berries.

2. Tofu Scramble Wrap:

   - Ingredients: Firm tofu, bell peppers, onions, spinach, turmeric, cumin, nutritional yeast, whole-grain tortilla.

   - Method: Sauté chopped vegetables, crumbled tofu, and spices until cooked. Fill a tortilla with the scramble for a protein-packed breakfast wrap.

3. Chickpea Flour Pancakes:

- Ingredients: Chickpea flour, water, baking powder, salt, vegetables (optional), avocado.

- Method: Mix chickpea flour, water, baking powder, and salt to make a batter. Cook as you would regular pancakes. Top with sautéed vegetables and sliced avocado.

4. Protein-Packed Smoothie Bowl:

- Ingredients: Frozen berries, banana, plant-based protein powder, almond milk, granola, chia seeds, sliced almonds.

- Method: Blend berries, banana, protein powder, and almond milk. Pour into a bowl and top with granola, chia seeds, and sliced almonds.

5. Lentil and Vegetable Breakfast Burrito:

- Ingredients: Cooked lentils, sautéed bell peppers and onions, avocado, whole-grain tortilla.

- Method: Combine cooked lentils and sautéed vegetables. Fill a tortilla, add sliced avocado, and wrap for a protein-rich breakfast burrito.

6. Quinoa Breakfast Bowl:

- Ingredients: Cooked quinoa, plant-based yogurt, mixed berries, nuts, seeds, drizzle of maple syrup.

- Method: Layer a bowl with quinoa and plant-based yogurt. Top with mixed berries, nuts, seeds, and a drizzle of maple syrup.

7. Vegan Protein Pancakes:

- Ingredients: Whole-grain flour, plant-based protein powder, almond milk, baking powder, vanilla extract.

- Method: Mix ingredients to make pancake batter. Cook on a griddle and serve with your favorite plant-based toppings.

8. Soy Yogurt Parfait:

- Ingredients: Soy yogurt, granola, sliced kiwi, chopped nuts.

- Method: Layer soy yogurt with granola, sliced kiwi, and chopped nuts to create a protein-packed parfait.

9. Chia Seed Pudding with Berries:

- Ingredients: Chia seeds, almond milk, vanilla extract, mixed berries.

- Method: Mix chia seeds, almond milk, and vanilla extract. Refrigerate until it forms a pudding-like consistency. Top with mixed berries.

10. Green Smoothie with Plant-Based Protein:

   - Ingredients: Spinach, kale, banana, plant-based protein powder, almond milk, chia seeds.

   - Method: Blend spinach, kale, banana, protein powder, and almond milk for a nutrient-dense green smoothie. Garnish with chia seeds.

Benefits of Plant-Based Protein Breakfasts

1. Sustained Energy: Plant-based proteins, combined with complex carbohydrates and healthy fats, provide sustained energy throughout the morning, reducing the likelihood of energy crashes.

2. Nutrient Density: Plant-based protein breakfasts are rich in essential nutrients, including fiber, vitamins, minerals, and antioxidants, contributing to overall well-being.

3. Digestive Health: The fiber content in many plant-based protein sources supports digestive health by promoting regular bowel movements and fostering a healthy gut microbiome.

4. Weight Management: Plant-based protein breakfasts can contribute to weight management by promoting feelings of fullness and reducing the likelihood of overeating later in the day.

5. Heart Health: Many plant-based protein sources are low in saturated fats and cholesterol, making them heart-healthy choices that may contribute to cardiovascular well-being.

6. Diverse Flavor Profiles: Plant-based proteins offer a wide range of flavors and textures, allowing for diverse and satisfying breakfast options to suit individual taste preferences.

Conclusion

Embracing a plant-based lifestyle doesn't mean sacrificing protein intake, especially at breakfast, the foundation of a productive day. The diverse plant-based protein breakfast ideas explored in this essay showcase the culinary possibilities that abound in the world of plant-powered nutrition. From savory tofu scrambles to sweet chia seed puddings, these breakfast options are not only rich in protein but also in flavor, providing a satisfying and nourishing start to the day.

As the demand for plant-based alternatives continues to grow, creative and delicious plant-based protein breakfasts are becoming more accessible and widely appreciated. Whether you're a seasoned plant-based enthusiast or someone looking to incorporate more plant-based options into your diet, these breakfast ideas offer a delightful and nutritious way to celebrate the power of plant-based proteins in fueling your mornings and supporting your overall well-being.

Lunch and Dinner Recipes

Plant-based living has surged in popularity, with an increasing number of individuals adopting a plant-centric approach to their dietary choices. Embracing a plant-based lifestyle doesn't mean compromising on taste, satisfaction, or nutritional value, particularly when it comes to lunch and dinner. In this essay, we'll explore a myriad of delicious and protein-packed lunch and dinner recipes that celebrate the versatility and goodness of plant-based proteins. From hearty bowls to savory stews and globally inspired dishes, these recipes showcase the bounty of plant-based ingredients that can delight the palate while nourishing the body.

The Essence of Plant-Based Proteins in Lunch and Dinner

Lunch and dinner serve as key opportunities to infuse a variety of plant-based proteins into one's diet, ensuring a well-rounded nutritional intake. Plant-based proteins play a vital role in supporting muscle health, providing essential amino acids, and contributing to overall satiety. As individuals explore the world of plant-based proteins, they discover the richness of options that extend beyond traditional meat-centric meals.

Key Plant-Based Protein Sources:

1. Legumes: Beans, lentils, chickpeas, and peas are excellent sources of plant-based proteins, offering a hearty and fiber-rich addition to a variety of dishes.

2. Tofu and Tempeh: Derived from soybeans, tofu and tempeh are versatile protein-packed options that absorb flavors well and lend themselves to various cooking methods.

3. Nuts and Seeds: Almonds, walnuts, chia seeds, flaxseeds, and hemp seeds contribute not only protein but also healthy fats, making them valuable additions to meals.

4. Whole Grains: Quinoa, brown rice, farro, and bulgur are whole grains that provide a combination of protein and complex carbohydrates for sustained energy.

5. Plant-Based Meat Alternatives: A variety of plant-based meat alternatives, made from ingredients like peas, soy, or wheat, offer familiar textures and flavors for those seeking alternatives to traditional meat.

Lunch and Dinner Recipes for Plant-Based Proteins

1. Chickpea and Spinach Curry:

   - Ingredients: Chickpeas, spinach, tomatoes, onions, garlic, ginger, curry spices, coconut milk.

   - Method: Sauté onions, garlic, and ginger. Add chickpeas, tomatoes, curry spices, and coconut milk. Simmer until flavors meld. Add spinach and cook until wilted. Serve over brown rice.

2. Quinoa and Black Bean Burrito Bowl:

   - Ingredients: Quinoa, black beans, corn, avocado, cherry tomatoes, lime, cilantro, salsa.

   - Method: Cook quinoa and black beans. Assemble a bowl with quinoa, black beans, corn, diced avocado, cherry tomatoes, cilantro, and a squeeze of lime. Top with salsa.

3. Vegan Lentil Bolognese:

   - Ingredients: Lentils, tomatoes, onions, garlic, carrots, celery, tomato paste, Italian herbs.

   - Method: Sauté onions, garlic, carrots, and celery. Add lentils, tomatoes, tomato paste, and herbs. Simmer until lentils are tender. Serve over whole-grain pasta.

4. Tofu Stir-Fry with Vegetables:

   - Ingredients: Firm tofu, broccoli, bell peppers, snap peas, carrots, soy sauce, ginger, garlic.

   - Method: Press and cube tofu. Sauté tofu until golden. Add vegetables, soy sauce, ginger, and garlic. Stir-fry until vegetables are tender. Serve over brown rice.

5. Mushroom and Walnut Stuffed Peppers:

   - Ingredients: Bell peppers, mushrooms, walnuts, quinoa, onions, garlic, tomato sauce.

   - Method: Sauté mushrooms, onions, and garlic. Add chopped walnuts and cooked quinoa. Stuff bell peppers with the mixture. Bake until peppers are tender. Top with tomato sauce.

6. Chickpea Salad Wraps:

   - Ingredients: Chickpeas, celery, red onion, vegan mayo, Dijon mustard, lettuce, whole-grain wraps.

   - Method: Mash chickpeas and mix with diced celery, red onion, vegan mayo, and Dijon mustard. Fill wraps with chickpea salad and lettuce.

7. Soy-Ginger Glazed Tempeh with Brown Rice:

   - Ingredients: Tempeh, soy sauce, ginger, garlic, maple syrup, brown rice.

   - Method: Marinate tempeh in a mixture of soy sauce, ginger, garlic, and maple syrup. Bake or pan-fry until golden. Serve over brown rice.

8. Vegan Mediterranean Bowl:

   - Ingredients: Quinoa, chickpeas, cucumber, cherry tomatoes, olives, red onion, hummus, lemon-tahini dressing.

   - Method: Assemble a bowl with quinoa, chickpeas, cucumber, cherry tomatoes, olives, and red onion. Drizzle with lemon-tahini dressing and top with hummus.

9. Stuffed Portobello Mushrooms with Spinach and Quinoa:

   - Ingredients: Portobello mushrooms, quinoa, spinach, garlic, onions, nutritional yeast.

   - Method: Remove mushroom stems and bake. Sauté onions, garlic, and spinach. Mix with cooked quinoa and stuff into mushrooms. Bake until mushrooms are tender.

10. Vegan Lentil Soup:

   - Ingredients: Lentils, carrots, celery, onions, garlic, vegetable broth, tomatoes, cumin, coriander.

   - Method: Sauté onions, garlic, carrots, and celery. Add lentils, tomatoes, vegetable broth, cumin, and coriander. Simmer until lentils are cooked. Serve as a comforting soup.

Benefits of Plant-Based Protein-Based Lunches and Dinners

1. Nutrient Density: Plant-based protein meals are rich in essential nutrients, including fiber, vitamins, minerals, and antioxidants, contributing to overall health.

2. Heart Health: Many plant-based protein sources are low in saturated fats and cholesterol, supporting cardiovascular well-being.

3. Weight Management: Plant-based proteins, combined with fiber-rich vegetables and whole grains, promote feelings of fullness, aiding in weight management.

4. Digestive Health: The fiber content in plant-based meals supports digestive health by promoting regular bowel movements and fostering a healthy gut microbiome.

5. Sustainable Eating: Plant-based proteins often have a lower environmental footprint compared to animal proteins, contributing to sustainable and eco-friendly dietary choices.

6. Diverse Flavor Profiles: Plant-based meals offer a wide range of flavors, textures, and global influences, creating a diverse and satisfying culinary experience.

Conclusion

Plant-based living has evolved from a niche choice to a mainstream culinary movement, and the lunch and dinner recipes explored in this essay exemplify the culinary delights that await those who embrace a plant-powered lifestyle. From the comforting lentil bolognese to the vibrant Mediterranean bowl, each recipe showcases the creativity and nourishment that plant-based proteins bring to the table.

As individuals continue to explore the diverse world of plant-based proteins, they not only discover the richness of flavors but also contribute to their overall health and well-being. Plant-based lunches and dinners go beyond the plate, representing a conscious choice for personal health, environmental sustainability, and culinary exploration. As we celebrate the beauty of plant-based proteins in our daily meals, we embark on a flavorful journey that nourishes the body, delights the palate, and supports a sustainable and compassionate way of living.

Snacks and On-the-Go Options

The realm of plant-based living extends far beyond traditional meals, reaching into the world of snacks and on-the-go options. As more individuals embrace plant-centric diets, the demand for convenient and protein-packed snacks has soared. This essay explores the diverse landscape of plant-based snacks and on-the-go options, showcasing the delicious and nutritious alternatives available for those seeking to infuse their day with the goodness of plant-based proteins. From portable bites to satisfying treats, these options demonstrate the versatility and accessibility of plant-powered protein.

The Rise of Plant-Based Snacking

Snacking has evolved from an occasional indulgence to a fundamental aspect of modern eating habits. Whether it's a mid-morning pick-me-up, an afternoon energy boost, or a pre-workout bite, snacks play a crucial role in sustaining energy levels throughout the day. The shift toward plant-based snacking aligns with broader trends in health-conscious and environmentally conscious consumer choices.

Key Plant-Based Protein Snack Sources:

1. Nuts and Seeds: Almonds, walnuts, chia seeds, flaxseeds, and hemp seeds are nutrient-dense and protein-rich options for snacking.

2. Legumes: Chickpeas, roasted edamame, and lentils can be seasoned and baked for a crunchy and satisfying snack.

3. Plant-Based Protein Bars: Bars made from ingredients like nuts, seeds, dried fruits, and plant-based protein powders provide a convenient on-the-go protein source.

4. Nut and Seed Butters: Spreadable options like almond butter, peanut butter, and sunflower seed butter can be paired with fruits or crackers for a quick and satiating snack.

5. Plant-Based Yogurts: Almond, soy, coconut, or oat-based yogurts offer a creamy and protein-packed snack base that can be customized with toppings.

6. Vegetables with Hummus or Guacamole: Sliced vegetables paired with hummus or guacamole provide a satisfying and nutrient-rich snack.

7. Roasted Chickpea Snacks: Chickpeas can be seasoned and roasted for a crunchy and protein-packed snack that comes in various flavors.

8. Protein-Packed Smoothies: Blending fruits, vegetables, plant-based protein powder, and plant-based milk creates a nutrient-rich and portable snack.

Plant-Based Protein Snack Ideas

1. Trail Mix with Nuts and Dried Fruits:

   - Ingredients: Almonds, walnuts, cashews, dried cranberries, raisins, dark chocolate chips.

   - Method: Mix the ingredients to create a balanced and protein-rich trail mix that can be portioned into snack-sized servings.

2. Chia Seed Pudding Parfait:

   - Ingredients: Chia seeds, almond milk, plant-based yogurt, mixed berries.

  - Method: Mix chia seeds with almond milk and refrigerate until it forms a pudding. Layer with plant-based yogurt and mixed berries for a parfait.

3. Roasted Chickpea Trio:

  - Ingredients: Canned chickpeas, olive oil, cumin, smoked paprika, garlic powder, sea salt.

  - Method: Season chickpeas and roast until crispy. Create three variations with different spice blends for a diverse and flavorful snack.

4. Apple Slices with Almond Butter:

  - Ingredients: Apples, almond butter.

  - Method: Slice apples and pair with almond butter for a satisfying and fiber-rich snack that combines natural sweetness with protein.

5. Veggie Sticks with Hummus:

  - Ingredients: Carrot sticks, cucumber slices, bell pepper strips, hummus.

  - Method: Slice vegetables and serve with hummus for a refreshing and crunchy snack that combines protein with vitamins and minerals.

6. Energy Bites with Oats and Nut Butter:

  - Ingredients: Rolled oats, nut butter, maple syrup, chia seeds, vanilla extract.

  - Method: Mix ingredients and roll into bite-sized balls. Refrigerate until firm, creating a convenient and energy-boosting snack.

7. Protein-Packed Smoothie Popsicles:

  - Ingredients: Mixed berries, plant-based protein powder, almond milk.

  - Method: Blend berries, protein powder, and almond milk. Pour into popsicle molds and freeze for a refreshing and protein-rich frozen treat.

8. Edamame Snack Bowl:

  - Ingredients: Roasted edamame, cherry tomatoes, avocado cubes, lime juice.

  - Method: Combine roasted edamame, cherry tomatoes, and avocado cubes. Drizzle with lime juice for a nutrient-packed snack bowl.

9. Plant-Based Protein Bars:

  - Ingredients (homemade): Dates, nuts, seeds, plant-based protein powder, dried fruits.

  - Method: Blend ingredients, press into a pan, and refrigerate until firm. Cut into bars for a homemade and customizable protein snack.

10. Vegan Yogurt Parfait Cup:

   - Ingredients: Plant-based yogurt, granola, sliced banana, berries.

   - Method: Layer plant-based yogurt with granola, sliced banana, and berries in a portable cup for an on-the-go parfait.

On-the-Go Plant-Based Protein Options

1. Roasted Chickpea Snack Packs:

   - Pre-packaged roasted chickpea snacks come in convenient single-serving packs, providing a portable and protein-rich option.

2. Nut and Seed Bars:

   - Store-bought nut and seed bars offer a quick and on-the-go source of plant-based protein, available in various flavors.

3. Protein-Packed Smoothie Bottles:

   - Pre-made protein smoothie bottles, often enriched with plant-based protein powder, are convenient options for a quick and nutritious on-the-go snack.

4. Individual Nut Butter Packets:

   - Single-serving packets of nut butter, such as almond or peanut butter, can be paired with fruits or crackers for a portable protein option.

5. Plant-Based Yogurt Cups:

   - Individual servings of plant-based yogurt cups are easily portable and can be enjoyed on their own or customized with toppings.

6. Dried Edamame Snack Packs:

   - Dried edamame snack packs offer a crunchy and protein-packed on-the-go option that requires no refrigeration.

7. Vegan Cheese and Crackers:

   - Pre-packaged vegan cheese and crackers provide a convenient and portable option for a protein-rich and savory snack.

8. Protein-Packed Energy Bars:

   - Various brands offer plant-based protein bars that cater to different dietary preferences, providing a quick and satisfying on-the-go option.

Benefits of Plant-Based Protein Snacks and On-the-Go Options

1. Convenience: Plant-based protein snacks and on-the-go options offer convenience for individuals with busy lifestyles, providing quick and easy access to protein-rich choices.

2. Sustained Energy: Combining plant-based proteins with fiber-rich ingredients in snacks supports sustained energy levels throughout the day, reducing the likelihood of energy crashes.

3. Nutrient Density: Plant-based protein snacks are often rich in essential nutrients, contributing not only to protein intake but also to overall health.

4. Satisfying and Flavorful: Plant-based snacks come in a variety of flavors and textures, satisfying cravings for both sweet and savory options.

5. Environmentally Friendly: Choosing plant-based snacks aligns with environmentally conscious choices, as plant-based protein sources typically have a lower environmental impact compared to animal-based options.

6. Diverse Options: The diversity of plant-based protein snacks allows individuals to explore and enjoy a wide range of flavors, cuisines, and culinary styles.

Conclusion

As the world of plant-based living continues to expand, so does the array of snacks and on-the-go options available to those seeking protein-packed alternatives. The recipes and ideas explored in this essay showcase the creativity and convenience inherent in plant-based protein snacks, demonstrating that nourishing choices can be both delicious and accessible.

Whether enjoying homemade energy bites, grabbing a pre-packaged protein bar, or savoring a yogurt parfait on the move, individuals embracing plant-based living have an abundance of options to fuel their day. The evolution of plant-based snacking not only caters to personal health and well-

being but also reflects a broader shift toward sustainable and mindful choices in the realm of nutrition. As we celebrate the power of plant-based proteins in snacks and on-the-go options, we embrace a flavorful and nourishing journey that complements the dynamic pace of modern life.

Chapter Four
Plant-Based Proteins In Diseases And Special Conditions

In recent years, the spotlight on plant-based nutrition has intensified as individuals seek healthier dietary choices that align with both personal well-being and environmental sustainability. Central to this dietary shift is the exploration of plant-based proteins and their impact on various diseases and special conditions. This essay delves into the nuanced relationship between plant-based proteins and health, examining their role in preventing, managing, and sometimes even mitigating the effects of specific diseases. From cardiovascular health to diabetes management, and considerations for special populations such as athletes and pregnant individuals, we explore the diverse implications of embracing plant-based protein sources.

Plant-based proteins form the cornerstone of plant-centric diets, encompassing a wide array of sources such as legumes, grains, nuts, seeds, and plant-based protein supplements. Unlike animal proteins, plant proteins may lack certain essential amino acids, necessitating strategic dietary planning to ensure a balanced amino acid profile. The versatility of plant-based proteins allows for a diverse and satisfying range of culinary options, making them accessible to a broad spectrum of individuals with varying dietary preferences.

Impact on Diseases:

1. Cardiovascular Diseases: Cardiovascular diseases (CVD) are a leading cause of morbidity and mortality globally. Plant-based diets, characterized by a higher intake of plant-based proteins, have been associated with a reduced risk of CVD.

- Cholesterol Management: Plant-based proteins, such as those found in legumes, nuts, and seeds, contribute to lower levels of low-density lipoprotein (LDL) cholesterol, often referred to as "bad" cholesterol. The absence of dietary cholesterol in plant-based proteins further supports heart health.

- Blood Pressure Control: The potassium-rich nature of many plant-based foods, combined with the blood pressure-lowering effects of plant-based proteins, contributes to better blood pressure control.

- Anti-Inflammatory Effects: Chronic inflammation is a key contributor to the development of atherosclerosis and heart disease. Plant-based proteins, with their anti-inflammatory properties, may help mitigate the inflammatory processes associated with CVD.

2. Diabetes Management: Diabetes, particularly type 2 diabetes, is a metabolic disorder characterized by impaired insulin function and elevated blood sugar levels. Plant-based diets, featuring plant-based proteins, have shown promise in managing diabetes.

- Fiber and Blood Sugar Control: The fiber content of plant-based diets, including plant-based proteins, plays a vital role in regulating blood sugar levels. Fiber slows down the absorption of glucose, contributing to better glycemic control.

- Improved Insulin Sensitivity: Plant-based diets have been linked to improved insulin sensitivity, which is crucial for individuals with diabetes. Plant-based proteins, in combination with other plant foods, support insulin function and glucose metabolism.

- Weight Management: Obesity is a significant risk factor for type 2 diabetes. Plant-based diets, supported by plant-based proteins, contribute to weight management and may reduce the risk of developing diabetes.

3. Cancer Prevention: The relationship between diet and cancer is complex, and while no single food can prevent cancer, plant-based diets with an emphasis on plant-based proteins may contribute to a lower risk of certain cancers.

- Antioxidant Protection: Plant-based proteins are often rich in antioxidants, which play a role in protecting cells from damage that could lead to cancer. Antioxidants neutralize free radicals, reducing the risk of cellular mutations.

- Phytochemicals and Cancer Protection: Plant foods, including those containing plant-based proteins, are sources of phytochemicals. These bioactive compounds have been studied for their potential protective effects against cancer development.

- Fiber and Digestive Health: Plant-based diets high in fiber, including fiber-rich plant-based proteins, contribute to healthy digestion. Adequate fiber intake is associated with a reduced risk of certain digestive cancers.

Plant-Based Proteins in Special Conditions:

1. Athletes and Physical Performance: Athletes have unique nutritional needs to support physical performance, muscle recovery, and overall well-being. The role of plant-based proteins in meeting these needs is a subject of growing interest.

- Adequate Protein Intake: Contrary to the misconception that plant-based diets lack sufficient protein for athletes, strategic planning allows individuals to meet their protein requirements through a combination of plant-based protein sources.

- Muscle Building and Recovery: Plant-based proteins, such as those found in legumes, tofu, tempeh, and plant-based protein supplements, offer essential amino acids necessary for muscle building and recovery.

- Anti-Inflammatory Effects: Intense physical activity can lead to inflammation. The anti-inflammatory properties of plant-based proteins contribute to faster recovery and reduced muscle soreness.

2. Pregnancy and Lactation: The nutritional needs during pregnancy and lactation are critical for the health of both the mother and the developing baby. Plant-based diets, when well-planned, can provide the necessary nutrients, including plant-based proteins.

- Protein for Fetal Development: Adequate protein intake is crucial for fetal development. Plant-based proteins from sources like legumes, whole grains, and nuts contribute to the protein requirements during pregnancy.

- Iron and Calcium Considerations: Plant-based diets may require special attention to ensure sufficient intake of iron and calcium, vital for the mother's health and the development of the baby's bones and teeth.

- Omega-3 Fatty Acids: Plant-based sources of omega-3 fatty acids, such as flaxseeds, chia seeds, and walnuts, can contribute to the essential fatty acids necessary for the baby's brain and eye development.

3. Childhood Nutrition: Plant-based diets can be suitable for children when carefully planned to meet their nutritional needs for growth and development. Attention to key nutrients, including protein, iron, calcium, and vitamin B12, is crucial.

- Protein Sources for Growth: Plant-based proteins, such as those from legumes, tofu, and plant-based dairy alternatives, can provide essential amino acids necessary for the growth and development of children.

- Diverse Nutrient Intake: Plant-based diets introduce children to a variety of nutrient-dense foods, promoting diverse nutrient intake and establishing healthy eating patterns.

- Supplementation Considerations: Depending on dietary choices and potential nutrient gaps, supplementation with vitamin B12 and other nutrients may be considered for children on plant-based diets.

4. Elderly Population: The nutritional needs of the elderly population differ from other age groups, and plant-based diets can be beneficial for promoting health and well-being in aging individuals.

- Protein for Muscle Health: Adequate protein intake is crucial for maintaining muscle mass, which tends to decline with age. Plant-based proteins contribute to overall protein needs in the elderly.

- Antioxidants and Cognitive Health: Plant-based diets, rich in antioxidants and anti-inflammatory compounds, may support cognitive health in aging individuals.

- Bone Health Considerations: Attention to calcium and vitamin D intake is important for maintaining bone health in the elderly. Plant-based sources, such as fortified plant milks and leafy greens, can contribute to these nutrients.

Challenges and Considerations:

While plant-based diets and proteins offer numerous health benefits, certain challenges and considerations merit attention:

1. Nutrient Deficiencies: Plant-based diets may be associated with certain nutrient deficiencies, such as vitamin B12, iron, calcium, and omega-3 fatty acids. Careful dietary planning, supplementation when necessary, and choosing fortified foods can address these concerns.

2. Protein Quality: While many plant-based proteins are high quality, some may lack specific amino acids. Combining different plant protein sources over the course of the day can ensure a balanced amino acid profile.

3. Digestibility: Some individuals may experience digestive discomfort with certain plant-based proteins. Soaking, fermenting, or cooking these foods can enhance digestibility.

4. Personalization of Diet: Nutritional needs vary among individuals, and there is no one-size-fits-all approach. Personalization of a plant-based diet based on individual health conditions, preferences, and cultural considerations is crucial.

Promoting Optimal Plant-Based Nutrition:

1. Diverse Protein Sources: Incorporating a variety of plant-based protein sources ensures a broad spectrum of nutrients and helps address potential gaps in amino acid profiles.

2. Whole Foods Emphasis: Prioritizing whole, minimally processed plant foods over highly processed alternatives contributes to overall health and maximizes nutrient intake.

3. Balanced Macronutrients: Ensuring a balance of macronutrients—protein, carbohydrates, and fats—supports overall health and helps meet energy requirements.

4. Supplementation When Necessary: In certain situations, supplementation with nutrients like vitamin B12, vitamin D, and omega-3 fatty acids may be necessary to address potential deficiencies.

5. Consultation with Healthcare Professionals: Individuals considering or adopting a plant-based diet, especially those with pre-existing health conditions, should consult with healthcare professionals or registered dietitians for personalized guidance.

Conclusion:

Plant-based proteins are integral to the promotion of health, the prevention of diseases, and the support of individuals with specific conditions. As the discourse around sustainable and health-conscious dietary choices intensifies, the integration of plant-based proteins into daily eating patterns emerges as a proactive step toward holistic well-being.

Navigating the complex interplay between plant-based proteins and diseases requires a nuanced understanding of individual health conditions, dietary preferences, and cultural considerations. By embracing the potential of plant-based proteins and adopting a mindful approach to dietary planning, individuals can harness the power of plant-based nutrition to foster a healthier and more sustainable world.

As research continues to unfold, highlighting the myriad benefits of plant-based diets and proteins, the landscape of nutrition is evolving. Through informed choices, thoughtful dietary planning, and ongoing collaboration between healthcare professionals and individuals, the journey toward optimal health and well-being becomes not only achievable but also deeply rewarding. In recognizing the integral role of plant-based proteins in diseases and special conditions, we embark on a path that not only nourishes the body but also sustains the planet for generations to come.

Chapter Five
Infants and Children

The dietary choices made during infancy and childhood play a crucial role in shaping long-term health outcomes. In recent years, there has been a growing interest in plant-based diets for children, emphasizing the incorporation of plant-based proteins to meet nutritional needs. This essay explores the role of plant-based proteins in the diet of infants and children, addressing the potential benefits, considerations, and strategies for ensuring optimal nutrition during these formative years.

The early years of life are characterized by rapid growth and development, making nutrition during infancy and childhood a critical factor in establishing a foundation for overall health. The choice of protein sources is particularly significant as proteins are essential for the building blocks of tissues, enzymes, hormones, and immune function. While traditional dietary guidelines have often centered around animal-based proteins, there is a growing recognition of the potential benefits of incorporating plant-based proteins into the diets of infants and children.

Plant-based proteins are derived from a variety of plant sources, including legumes, grains, nuts, seeds, and plant-based protein products. Unlike animal proteins, plant-based proteins may lack certain essential amino acids, requiring attention to dietary variety to ensure a complete amino acid profile. The inclusion of a diverse array of plant-based protein sources allows for the provision of essential nutrients and micronutrients crucial for growth and development.

Nutritional Requirements in Infancy:

Infancy is a period of rapid growth and development, and meeting specific nutritional requirements is paramount for ensuring optimal health. Key nutritional considerations during infancy include:

1. Protein Needs: Infants require an adequate intake of protein to support the development of muscles, organs, and tissues. While breast milk or formula is the primary source of nutrition during the first year of life, the introduction of complementary foods marks the beginning of exposure to various protein sources.

2. Energy Requirements: Meeting energy needs is essential for growth and development. Adequate energy intake supports not only physical growth but also cognitive development during infancy.

3. Micronutrients: Infants have specific requirements for essential micronutrients such as iron, zinc, calcium, vitamin D, and omega-3 fatty acids. These nutrients are crucial for the development of bones, immune function, and cognitive processes.

Benefits of Plant-Based Proteins for Infants:

1. Diverse Nutrient Profile: Plant-based proteins bring a diverse array of nutrients, including fiber, vitamins, minerals, and antioxidants. Exposure to a variety of plant foods broadens the nutrient intake of infants, contributing to overall health.

2. Gentle Introduction to Solid Foods: As infants transition from a liquid diet (breast milk or formula) to solid foods, plant-based proteins offer a gentle introduction. Plant-based sources, such as mashed legumes, pureed vegetables, and cereals, provide texture and flavor diversity.

3. Reduced Risk of Food Allergies: Introducing a variety of plant-based proteins early in life may be associated with a reduced risk of developing food allergies. Delaying the introduction of allergenic foods, including certain plant-based proteins, has been suggested as a strategy to lower allergy risk.

4. Establishing Healthy Eating Patterns: Introducing plant-based proteins in infancy contributes to the establishment of healthy eating patterns. Early exposure to a variety of flavors and textures from plant foods fosters an appreciation for diverse foods later in life.

Plant-Based Proteins in Childhood:

As children transition from infancy to childhood, their nutritional needs continue to evolve. The incorporation of plant-based proteins remains a valuable component of a well-balanced diet, offering specific benefits in childhood:

1. Growth and Development: Plant-based proteins provide essential amino acids necessary for the ongoing growth and development of children. Sources such as legumes, tofu, and whole grains contribute to the protein needs required for muscle development and overall growth.

2. Cognitive Function: Nutrients found in plant-based proteins, including omega-3 fatty acids, vitamins, and minerals, play a role in supporting cognitive function. These nutrients are essential for brain development and academic achievement.

3. Healthy Weight Maintenance: Plant-based diets, when balanced and varied, contribute to healthy weight maintenance in children. The fiber content of plant foods promotes satiety, reducing the likelihood of excessive calorie intake.

4. Reduced Risk of Chronic Diseases: The establishment of healthy eating patterns centered around plant-based proteins in childhood may contribute to a reduced risk of chronic diseases later in life. Plant-based diets have been associated with a lower risk of obesity, type 2 diabetes, and cardiovascular diseases.

Considerations for Optimal Nutrition:

While plant-based diets can offer numerous benefits, certain considerations are crucial for ensuring optimal nutrition in infants and children:

1. Complete Protein Intake: Plant-based proteins may lack specific essential amino acids found in animal proteins. To ensure a complete amino acid profile, it is essential to offer a variety of plant-based protein sources, combining complementary proteins throughout the day.

2. Iron and Zinc Absorption: Plant-based sources of iron (non-heme iron) and zinc may have lower absorption rates compared to their animal-based counterparts. Including vitamin C-rich foods in meals enhances the absorption of non-heme iron, while incorporating zinc-rich plant foods is essential for zinc intake.

3. Omega-3 Fatty Acids: Omega-3 fatty acids, crucial for brain development, are found in certain plant sources such as flaxseeds, chia seeds, and walnuts. Including these foods in the diet contributes to a sufficient intake of essential fatty acids.

4. Calcium Needs: Plant-based sources of calcium, including fortified plant milks, leafy greens, and tofu, should be included to support bone health. Adequate vitamin D intake, either through sunlight exposure or supplementation, is essential for calcium absorption.

5. Supplementation When Necessary: Depending on dietary choices and potential nutrient gaps, supplementation with vitamin B12, vitamin D, and omega-3 fatty acids may be considered. Regular monitoring of growth and development, along with blood tests, can guide appropriate supplementation.

Plant-Based Protein Sources for Infants and Children:

1. Breast Milk or Formula (0-12 Months): Breast milk or formula provides the primary source of nutrition for infants during the first year of life. Breast milk, in particular, offers a complete and balanced profile of nutrients, including proteins, fats, and carbohydrates.

2. Legumes: Lentils, chickpeas, black beans, and other legumes are excellent sources of plant-based proteins for children. They can be introduced as purees, mashed, or included in soups and stews.

3. Tofu and Tempeh: Tofu and tempeh are soy-based products that provide high-quality plant-based proteins. They can be incorporated into various dishes, such as stir-fries, sandwiches, and salads.

4. Whole Grains: Whole grains like quinoa, brown rice, oats, and barley offer a source of plant-based proteins. These grains can be introduced as part of cereals, porridges, or side dishes.

5. Nuts and Seeds: Almonds, walnuts, chia seeds, and flaxseeds are rich in plant-based proteins, healthy fats, and essential nutrients. Nut butters can be introduced as spreads or additions to smoothies.

6. Plant-Based Dairy Alternatives: Fortified plant milks, such as almond milk, soy milk, and oat milk, can be included to provide calcium and vitamin D. Ensure that these alternatives are fortified to meet nutritional needs.

7. Vegetables: Some vegetables, such as broccoli and spinach, contain notable amounts of plant-based proteins. Incorporating a variety of vegetables in the diet ensures a diverse nutrient intake.

Educational and Culinary Approaches:

1. Nutrition Education: Parental education on the nutritional needs of infants and children on plant-based diets is essential. Understanding the importance of a balanced and varied diet, as well as potential nutrient gaps, enables parents to make informed choices.

2. Introduction of Diverse Flavors: Introducing a variety of flavors from plant-based foods early in infancy contributes to the development of a diverse palate. Exposing children to different tastes fosters an appreciation for a wide range of foods.

3. Involvement in Food Preparation: Involving children in the preparation of meals can enhance their interest in plant-based foods. Cooking together as a family promotes a positive attitude toward food and encourages healthy eating habits.

4. Plant-Based Recipes for Children: Exploring and creating plant-based recipes tailored to the preferences of children can make the dining experience enjoyable. Plant-based versions of familiar dishes, such as veggie burgers, plant-based pizza, and pasta with vegetable-based sauces, can be appealing to children.

Challenges and Solutions:

1. Protein Quality: Ensuring the quality of plant-based proteins may require a combination of different sources to achieve a complete amino acid profile. Combining legumes with grains, nuts, and seeds over the course of the day addresses this challenge.

2. Iron and Zinc Absorption: Plant-based sources of iron and zinc may have lower bioavailability. Enhancing the absorption of non-heme iron by pairing iron-rich plant foods with vitamin C-rich foods and including zinc-rich plant sources helps overcome this challenge.

3. Calcium Intake: Meeting calcium needs without relying on dairy products may require careful selection of fortified plant milks and other calcium-rich plant foods. Attention to vitamin D intake is essential for calcium absorption.

4. B12 Supplementation: Vitamin B12, primarily found in animal products, may require supplementation for individuals on strict plant-based diets. Regular monitoring and B12 supplementation, as recommended by healthcare professionals, address this concern.

Conclusion:

Plant-based proteins play a vital role in the nutrition of infants and children, contributing to growth, development, and overall well-being. The inclusion of diverse plant-based protein sources offers a rich array of nutrients, promoting a foundation for a lifetime of healthy eating habits. As dietary patterns evolve and awareness of the environmental and ethical aspects of food choices grows, plant-based nutrition for infants and children represents a thoughtful and sustainable approach.

Parental guidance, education, and culinary creativity are integral components in ensuring the successful integration of plant-based proteins into the diets of infants and children. By addressing potential challenges and leveraging the nutritional benefits of plant-based foods, caregivers can provide a nourishing environment that supports the health and development of the next generation.

In navigating the complex landscape of childhood nutrition, embracing the potential of plant-based proteins emerges as a proactive step toward fostering not only individual health but also a sustainable and compassionate relationship with food. As research continues to shed light on the intricacies of plant-based nutrition in infancy and childhood, the opportunity to optimize health outcomes for the next generation becomes increasingly achievable. In nurturing children with a plant-powered foundation, we contribute to a future where health, environmental consciousness, and ethical considerations harmoniously coexist.

Adolescents and Adults

As the awareness of health, environmental sustainability, and ethical considerations continues to grow, plant-based diets have gained prominence among adolescents and adults. Central to the success of plant-based nutrition is the incorporation of plant-based proteins, which serve as essential building blocks for maintaining health and well-being. This essay explores the role of plant-based proteins in the diets of adolescents and adults, examining the potential benefits, nutritional considerations, and broader implications for personal and planetary health.

Adolescence is a pivotal stage marked by rapid growth, hormonal changes, and the development of lifelong habits. Nutrition during this period plays a critical role in supporting physical and cognitive development, laying the foundation for future health. The inclusion of plant-based proteins in the diet of adolescents offers unique advantages and considerations.

Benefits of Plant-Based Proteins in Adolescence:

1. Growth and Development: Adequate protein intake is crucial during adolescence to support the growth and development of muscles, bones, and organs. Plant-based proteins, derived from sources such as legumes, tofu, and whole grains, provide essential amino acids necessary for these processes.

2. Nutrient Diversity: Plant-based proteins come with a diverse array of accompanying nutrients, including fiber, vitamins, minerals, and antioxidants. This nutrient diversity contributes to overall health and ensures adolescents receive a wide spectrum of essential nutrients.

3. Establishing Lifelong Habits: Adolescence is a formative period for establishing dietary habits that often persist into adulthood. Introducing and embracing plant-based proteins during this stage fosters a positive attitude toward plant-centric eating, promoting long-term health.

4. Sustainable Eating Habits: The ethical and environmental dimensions of food choices become increasingly relevant during adolescence. Choosing plant-based proteins aligns with sustainability goals, as plant agriculture generally has a lower environmental impact compared to animal agriculture.

Nutritional Considerations for Adolescents:

1. Protein Quality: While plant-based proteins may lack certain essential amino acids found in animal proteins, the quality of plant proteins can be optimized through a diverse and well-balanced diet. Combining different plant protein sources ensures a complete amino acid profile.

2. Caloric Needs: Adolescents experience a surge in energy requirements due to growth spurts and increased physical activity. Plant-based diets, rich in nutrient-dense foods, help meet these caloric needs while providing essential nutrients.

3. Iron and Calcium Intake: Plant-based sources of iron (non-heme iron) and calcium may have lower absorption rates compared to their animal-based counterparts. Including vitamin C-rich foods with iron-rich plant sources enhances iron absorption, and attention to calcium-rich plant foods supports bone health.

4. Educational Support:Nutrition education plays a crucial role in ensuring adolescents understand the importance of balanced plant-based nutrition. Providing resources and information empowers adolescents to make informed food choices that align with their health and ethical values.

Adulthood: Navigating Plant-Based Proteins for Health and Sustainability

As individuals transition into adulthood, the choices they make regarding nutrition profoundly impact their health and well-being. Plant-based proteins offer a sustainable and health-conscious approach to dietary habits in adulthood, addressing various health concerns while contributing to environmental stewardship.

Health Benefits of Plant-Based Proteins in Adulthood:

1. Heart Health: Plant-based diets, supported by plant-based proteins, have been associated with improved heart health. The lower saturated fat content and higher fiber intake contribute to lower cholesterol levels and reduced risk of cardiovascular diseases.

2. Weight Management: Plant-based diets, when focused on whole, minimally processed foods, are often associated with weight management. The fiber content of plant foods contributes to feelings of fullness, potentially reducing overall calorie intake.

3. Blood Sugar Control: Plant-based diets, particularly those emphasizing complex carbohydrates and plant-based proteins, have shown positive effects on blood sugar control. The fiber content helps stabilize blood glucose levels.

4. Cancer Prevention: While the relationship between diet and cancer is complex, plant-based diets with an emphasis on plant-based proteins have been associated with a lower risk of certain cancers. Antioxidants and phytochemicals found in plant foods may play a protective role.

5. Gut Health: Plant-based diets rich in fiber promote gut health by supporting a diverse and healthy microbiome. A healthy gut microbiome is linked to various aspects of overall health, including immune function and mental well-being.

Considerations for Plant-Based Nutrition in Adulthood:

1. Protein Intake for Muscle Health: Maintaining muscle mass becomes increasingly important in adulthood. Plant-based proteins, such as those found in legumes, tofu, and plant-based protein supplements, provide essential amino acids necessary for muscle health.

2. Bone Health and Calcium: Attention to calcium intake remains crucial for bone health in adulthood. Plant-based sources, including fortified plant milks, leafy greens, and tofu, can contribute to calcium needs.

3. Omega-3 Fatty Acids: Plant-based sources of omega-3 fatty acids, such as flaxseeds, chia seeds, and walnuts, play a role in supporting heart health and cognitive function. Including these foods in the diet contributes to an adequate intake of essential fatty acids.

4. B12 Supplementation: Vitamin B12, primarily found in animal products, may require supplementation for individuals on strict plant-based diets. Regular monitoring and B12 supplementation, as recommended by healthcare professionals, address this concern.

5. Whole Foods Emphasis: Emphasizing whole, minimally processed plant foods over highly processed alternatives supports overall health and maximizes nutrient intake. This approach also aligns with sustainability goals by reducing reliance on heavily processed foods.

Sustainability and Ethical Considerations:

1. Environmental Impact: Plant-based diets generally have a lower environmental footprint compared to diets centered around animal products. Reduced land use, water consumption, and greenhouse gas emissions contribute to the overall sustainability of plant-based eating.

2. Ethical Choices: Plant-based diets align with ethical considerations related to animal welfare. Choosing plant-based proteins reflects a commitment to compassionate and cruelty-free food choices, resonating with individuals who prioritize ethical treatment of animals.

3. Global Food Security: Plant-based diets are often viewed as a sustainable solution to global food security challenges. The efficient conversion of plant-based proteins into edible calories, compared to the resource-intensive production of animal proteins, supports the potential for equitable and sustainable food systems.

Culinary Exploration and Lifestyle Integration:

1. Diverse Plant-Based Recipes: The exploration of diverse plant-based recipes enhances the culinary experience for adults. Plant-based proteins can be incorporated into a variety of dishes, including salads, stir-fries, curries, and plant-based protein bowls.

2. Cultural Adaptation: Integrating plant-based proteins into various cultural cuisines allows individuals to maintain dietary practices rooted in tradition while embracing plant-centric choices. Adapting plant-based proteins to familiar recipes ensures a seamless transition to a plant-based lifestyle.

3. Restaurant and Social Options: The growing popularity of plant-based diets has led to increased options in restaurants and social settings. Individuals can now find a wide range of plant-based protein sources when dining out, making plant-based eating more accessible and enjoyable.

4. Education and Cooking Skills: Developing cooking skills and gaining knowledge about plant-based nutrition empower adults to make informed choices. Educational initiatives, cooking classes, and resources on plant-based cooking facilitate the integration of plant-based proteins into daily life.

Challenges and Solutions in Adulthood:

1. Nutrient Deficiencies: Adulthood brings the potential for nutrient deficiencies, especially in vitamin B12, iron, calcium, and omega-3 fatty acids. Regular monitoring, strategic dietary planning, and supplementation when necessary address these concerns.

2. Social and Cultural Influences: Social and cultural factors can influence dietary choices in adulthood. Addressing potential challenges related to social gatherings, cultural expectations, and peer influences requires open communication and proactive planning.

3. Balancing Macronutrients: Ensuring a balance of macronutrients—protein, carbohydrates, and fats—supports overall health. Balancing plant-based proteins with a variety of whole foods contributes to a well-rounded and satisfying diet.

4. Personalization of Diet: Individual dietary needs and preferences vary, and there is no one-size-fits-all approach to plant-based nutrition. Personalizing a plant-based diet based on individual health conditions, cultural considerations, and taste preferences is key.

Conclusion:

Plant-based proteins play a central role in the health and sustainability of adolescents and adults. As individuals navigate the complexities of dietary choices, embracing plant-based proteins emerges as a proactive and conscious decision with far-reaching implications. From supporting growth and development in adolescence to promoting heart health and sustainability in adulthood, the benefits of plant-based proteins extend across the lifespan.

Navigating the multifaceted landscape of plant-based nutrition in adolescence and adulthood requires a holistic approach that considers health, ethical considerations, and environmental impact. By embracing plant-based proteins, individuals contribute not only to their personal well-being but also to the broader goals of creating a sustainable and compassionate food system.

As research continues to evolve and awareness grows, the integration of plant-based proteins into everyday eating patterns becomes an integral aspect of health-conscious and environmentally responsible living. The journey toward optimal health, ethical choices, and sustainability is a dynamic and evolving process—one in which plant-based proteins play a vital and transformative role. In making informed choices, fostering culinary exploration, and embracing the broader implications of plant-based nutrition, individuals embark on a path that not only nourishes their own well-being but also contributes to a more sustainable and compassionate world.

Seniors

As individuals transition into their senior years, maintaining optimal health becomes a paramount concern. Nutrition plays a pivotal role in the well-being of seniors, influencing factors such as cognitive function, bone health, and overall vitality. Embracing a plant-based diet, rich in plant-based proteins, offers a holistic approach to senior nutrition, addressing the unique needs and challenges that come with aging. This essay delves into the significance of plant-based proteins in the diets of seniors, exploring the potential benefits, nutritional considerations, and strategies for promoting health and vitality in the golden years.

The Aging Process and Nutritional Needs:

The aging process is accompanied by physiological changes that impact nutrient absorption, metabolism, and overall health. Seniors often face challenges such as reduced muscle mass, diminished bone density, and a higher susceptibility to chronic diseases. Nutrition plays a crucial role in mitigating these challenges and promoting a higher quality of life during the aging process.

Benefits of Plant-Based Proteins for Seniors:

1. Muscle Maintenance and Strength: Maintaining muscle mass is particularly important for seniors to support mobility and overall strength. Plant-based proteins, including those from legumes, tofu, and nuts, provide essential amino acids necessary for muscle health.

2. Bone Health and Calcium Intake: Osteoporosis and bone fractures become more prevalent in seniors, emphasizing the importance of calcium intake. Plant-based sources of calcium, such as fortified plant milks, leafy greens, and tofu, contribute to bone health.

3. Heart Health: Seniors often face an increased risk of cardiovascular diseases. Plant-based diets, with their lower saturated fat content, have been associated with improved heart health, contributing to the prevention of heart-related issues.

4. Digestive Health and Fiber: Maintaining digestive health is crucial for seniors, and plant-based diets rich in fiber support regular bowel movements and prevent constipation. Fiber also aids in the management of cholesterol levels and promotes a healthy gut microbiome.

5. Anti-Inflammatory Effects: Chronic inflammation is associated with various age-related diseases. Plant-based proteins, abundant in antioxidants and anti-inflammatory compounds, contribute to reducing inflammation and supporting overall well-being.

Nutritional Considerations for Seniors:

1. Protein Intake for Muscle Health: The importance of protein intake for muscle health is heightened in seniors. Plant-based proteins, when combined in a well-balanced and varied diet, can meet these needs and contribute to maintaining muscle mass.

2. Calcium and Vitamin D: Adequate calcium and vitamin D intake is crucial for bone health. Plant-based sources of calcium, along with sunlight exposure for vitamin D synthesis, are essential components of a senior's diet.

3. B12 Supplementation: Vitamin B12 absorption tends to decrease with age, and seniors on plant-based diets may require supplementation. Regular monitoring and B12 supplementation, as recommended by healthcare professionals, address this concern.

4. Iron and Zinc Intake: Plant-based sources of iron (non-heme iron) and zinc may have lower absorption rates compared to animal-based sources. Including vitamin C-rich foods with iron-rich plant sources enhances iron absorption, and attention to zinc-rich plant foods supports overall health.

5. Omega-3 Fatty Acids: Omega-3 fatty acids play a role in cognitive health and cardiovascular function. Plant-based sources, such as flaxseeds, chia seeds, and walnuts, contribute to the essential fatty acids necessary for seniors.

Cognitive Health and Plant-Based Proteins:

Cognitive health is a significant concern for seniors, with conditions such as dementia and Alzheimer's disease posing challenges to independence and quality of life. Plant-based diets, rich in antioxidants and neuroprotective compounds, have been studied for their potential impact on cognitive function.

1. Antioxidants and Neuroprotection: Plant-based foods are abundant in antioxidants, which have neuroprotective properties. These compounds may help reduce oxidative stress and inflammation in the brain, contributing to cognitive health.

2. Omega-3 Fatty Acids: Plant-based sources of omega-3 fatty acids, including alpha-linolenic acid (ALA), contribute to brain health. These fatty acids play a role in maintaining cognitive function and may have protective effects against age-related cognitive decline.

3. Flavonoids and Polyphenols: Plant-based foods, such as berries, tea, and dark leafy greens, contain flavonoids and polyphenols with potential cognitive benefits. These compounds may enhance memory and support overall brain function.

4. Blood Sugar Control: Plant-based diets, particularly those focused on whole, minimally processed foods, contribute to stable blood sugar levels. Blood sugar control is crucial for reducing the risk of cognitive decline and dementia.

Challenges and Considerations for Seniors:

1. Digestive Issues: Seniors may experience digestive issues, such as decreased stomach acid production and slower digestion. Cooking methods that enhance the digestibility of plant-based foods, such as steaming and blending, can be beneficial.

2. Appetite and Taste Changes: Changes in appetite and taste perception are common in seniors. Adapting plant-based recipes to incorporate a variety of flavors and textures can make meals more appealing and enjoyable.

3. Social and Cultural Factors: Social and cultural factors can influence dietary choices in seniors. Addressing potential challenges related to social gatherings, cultural expectations, and peer influences requires open communication and proactive planning.

4. Medication Interactions: Some plant-based foods may interact with medications commonly taken by seniors. Healthcare professionals should be consulted to ensure that plant-based diets are compatible with existing medication regimens.

Strategies for Promoting Plant-Based Nutrition in Seniors:

1. Educational Initiatives: Implementing educational initiatives that emphasize the benefits of plant-based nutrition for seniors can empower them to make informed dietary choices. Workshops, seminars, and informational materials can play a crucial role in disseminating knowledge.

2. Culinary Exploration and Cooking Classes: Encouraging seniors to participate in cooking classes and culinary exploration can enhance their interest in plant-based foods. Learning new recipes and cooking techniques fosters a positive attitude toward plant-based nutrition.

3. Meal Planning Assistance: Providing meal planning assistance, including pre-prepared plant-based meals or meal kit services, can alleviate the burden of cooking for seniors. This ensures that they have access to nutritious and convenient plant-based options.

4. Collaboration with Healthcare Professionals: Collaboration with healthcare professionals, including dietitians and nutritionists, is essential to tailor plant-based diets to the specific health needs of seniors. Regular check-ups and nutritional assessments help monitor the impact of plant-based nutrition on overall health.

5. Community Engagement: Creating a sense of community around plant-based nutrition can offer support and encouragement for seniors. Group activities, shared meals, and community gardens foster a supportive environment for embracing plant-based lifestyles.

Social and Environmental Benefits:

1. Reduced Environmental Impact: Plant-based diets have a lower environmental footprint compared to diets centered around animal products. Seniors can contribute to sustainability efforts by choosing plant-based proteins, aligning with a broader commitment to environmental responsibility.

2. Ethical Considerations: Choosing plant-based proteins reflects a commitment to ethical considerations, including animal welfare. Seniors who prioritize ethical treatment of animals can align their dietary choices with their values.

3. Healthier Aging and Independence: The adoption of plant-based diets contributes to healthier aging, promoting independence and an enhanced quality of life for seniors. Maintaining physical and cognitive health supports autonomy and active living in the senior years.

Conclusion:

In the golden years of life, plant-based proteins emerge as a cornerstone for promoting health, well-being, and vitality among seniors. The benefits of plant-based nutrition extend beyond the individual, encompassing cognitive health, bone density, and the potential for healthier aging. As seniors navigate the complexities of aging, embracing plant-based proteins offers a proactive and conscious approach to nutrition that aligns with individual health goals, ethical considerations, and environmental stewardship.

By addressing the unique nutritional needs of seniors, considering potential challenges, and implementing strategies for promoting plant-based nutrition, individuals can experience the transformative impact of plant-based diets in their later years. Nurturing health and well-being through the consumption of plant-based proteins not only enhances the quality of life for seniors but also contributes to a more sustainable and compassionate approach to nutrition.

As the understanding of senior nutrition evolves and awareness grows, the integration of plant-based proteins into the dietary landscape of seniors becomes an integral aspect of promoting health and vitality in the golden years. By fostering a culture of informed choices, culinary exploration, and community support, seniors can embrace plant-based nutrition as a lifelong companion on their journey towards healthier and more fulfilling aging.

Chapter Six
Balancing Macronutrients

In the pursuit of optimal health and well-being, the concept of balancing macronutrients has gained prominence as a fundamental aspect of nutrition. Macronutrients—carbohydrates, proteins, and fats—serve as the primary sources of energy for the body, influencing various physiological functions. Achieving a harmonious balance of these macronutrients is not merely a dietary strategy; it is a cornerstone for supporting metabolic health, preventing nutritional imbalances, and promoting overall vitality. This essay explores the importance of balancing macronutrients, the role of each macronutrient in the body, and practical strategies for achieving a well-rounded and nutritious diet.

Understanding Macronutrients: The Building Blocks of Nutrition

Macronutrients are nutrients that the body requires in relatively large quantities to sustain life and support various physiological functions. They provide the energy needed for everyday activities and serve as essential building blocks for the body's structural components. Let's delve into the distinctive roles of each macronutrient:

1. Carbohydrates: Carbohydrates are the body's primary source of energy. They consist of sugars, starches, and fibers, which are broken down into glucose—a form of sugar that the body uses for fuel. Carbohydrates are found in various foods, including fruits, vegetables, grains, legumes, and dairy products.

   - Simple Carbohydrates: These are sugars that are quickly absorbed by the body and provide a rapid source of energy. Examples include table sugar, honey, and the natural sugars found in fruits (fructose) and milk (lactose).

   - Complex Carbohydrates: These are longer chains of sugars that take longer to break down, providing a more sustained release of energy. Foods rich in complex carbohydrates include whole grains, legumes, and vegetables.

Carbohydrates play a crucial role in supporting physical activity, brain function, and overall metabolic health. Balancing the types and amounts of carbohydrates in the diet is essential for maintaining stable blood sugar levels and preventing energy fluctuations.

2. Proteins: Proteins are essential for building and repairing tissues, supporting immune function, and serving as enzymes and hormones. Proteins are composed of amino acids, which are the building blocks that the body needs for various physiological processes. Dietary sources

of protein include meat, poultry, fish, dairy products, eggs, legumes, and plant-based sources such as tofu and tempeh.

- Essential Amino Acids: These are amino acids that the body cannot produce on its own and must be obtained through the diet. Foods that contain all essential amino acids are considered complete proteins and are often found in animal sources.

- Non-Essential Amino Acids: These are amino acids that the body can produce on its own. Foods that lack one or more essential amino acids are considered incomplete proteins and are often found in plant-based sources.

Balancing protein intake is crucial for maintaining muscle mass, supporting immune function, and promoting overall health. Adequate protein intake becomes particularly important during periods of growth, such as childhood and adolescence, as well as in situations where the body is repairing tissues, such as during recovery from illness or injury.

3. Fats: Fats, also known as lipids, are essential for various physiological functions, including cell structure, hormone production, and the absorption of fat-soluble vitamins (A, D, E, K). While fats have long been associated with concerns about weight gain, it's important to recognize the role of healthy fats in supporting overall health. Dietary sources of fats include oils, nuts, seeds, avocados, fatty fish, and dairy products.

- Saturated Fats: Found in animal products and some tropical oils, saturated fats are often considered less healthful when consumed in excess. However, they play a role in hormone production and cell structure.

- Monounsaturated Fats: Found in olive oil, avocados, and nuts, monounsaturated fats are associated with heart health and may have anti-inflammatory properties.

- Polyunsaturated Fats: Omega-3 and Omega-6 fatty acids, both polyunsaturated fats, are essential for the body and must be obtained through the diet. Fatty fish, flaxseeds, chia seeds, and walnuts are rich sources of omega-3 fatty acids.

Balancing the types of fats consumed and moderating overall fat intake is key to promoting heart health, supporting brain function, and ensuring the absorption of fat-soluble vitamins.

The Importance of Balancing Macronutrients:

Balancing macronutrients is not a one-size-fits-all approach but rather a dynamic process that considers individual factors such as age, sex, activity level, and health status. Several key aspects underscore the importance of achieving a harmonious balance of macronutrients:

1. Energy Balance: Balancing macronutrients is integral to achieving and maintaining energy balance. Consuming an appropriate amount of calories from carbohydrates, proteins, and fats

ensures that the body's energy needs are met without excessive caloric intake, preventing weight gain.

2. Blood Sugar Regulation: Carbohydrates play a crucial role in regulating blood sugar levels. Balancing the intake of carbohydrates with proteins and fats helps prevent sharp spikes and crashes in blood sugar, promoting stable energy levels and reducing the risk of insulin resistance.

3. Muscle Maintenance and Growth: Adequate protein intake is essential for muscle maintenance and growth. Balancing protein intake with carbohydrates and fats supports muscle protein synthesis, contributing to overall strength and preventing muscle wasting.

4. Hormone Production: Fats are crucial for hormone production, including hormones that regulate metabolism, reproductive function, and stress response. Balancing fat intake with other macronutrients supports hormonal balance, influencing various physiological processes.

5. Nutrient Absorption: Macronutrients play a role in the absorption of micronutrients. For example, some vitamins (e.g., vitamin D) are fat-soluble and require dietary fats for proper absorption. A well-balanced diet ensures optimal nutrient absorption and utilization.

Strategies for Balancing Macronutrients:

Achieving a balanced intake of macronutrients involves mindful dietary choices and an understanding of individual nutritional needs. Several practical strategies can help individuals achieve and maintain a well-rounded and nutritious diet:

1. Diverse Food Choices: Consuming a variety of foods from different food groups ensures a diverse intake of macronutrients and micronutrients. Incorporate a rainbow of fruits, vegetables, whole grains, and proteins into meals to maximize nutrient diversity.

2. Portion Control: Paying attention to portion sizes helps prevent overconsumption of any particular macronutrient. Using visual cues, such as the palm of the hand, to estimate appropriate serving sizes for proteins, carbohydrates, and fats can be a helpful strategy.

3. Mindful Eating: Practicing mindful eating involves being present and attentive during meals. This approach encourages listening to hunger and fullness cues, preventing overeating and promoting a balanced intake of macronutrients.

4. Macronutrient Ratios: While individual macronutrient needs vary, adopting a balanced macronutrient ratio can serve as a general guideline. For example, a balanced meal might include a mix of carbohydrates (e.g., whole grains), proteins (e.g., lean meats or plant-based proteins), and healthy fats (e.g., avocados or olive oil).

5. Consider Individual Needs: Individual nutritional needs vary based on factors such as age, gender, activity level, and health conditions. Consulting with a registered dietitian or nutritionist can provide personalized guidance to tailor macronutrient intake to individual requirements.

The Interplay of Macronutrients in Health and Disease:

Understanding the interplay of macronutrients goes beyond the context of a balanced diet; it extends to their impact on health and the prevention of chronic diseases. Different dietary patterns, such as vegetarianism, veganism, or low-carbohydrate diets, underscore the diverse ways in which macronutrients can be configured to support specific health goals.

1. Vegetarian and Vegan Diets: Vegetarian and vegan diets, which focus on plant-based sources of macronutrients, have gained popularity for their potential health benefits. These diets are rich in fiber, antioxidants, and phytochemicals, contributing to improved heart health and reduced inflammation. However, attention is needed to ensure adequate intake of nutrients that may be less abundant in plant-based sources, such as vitamin B12, iron, zinc, and omega-3 fatty acids.

2. Low-Carb and Ketogenic Diets: Low-carbohydrate and ketogenic diets restrict carbohydrate intake and emphasize higher fat consumption. These dietary patterns have been associated with weight loss, improved insulin sensitivity, and cardiovascular benefits. However, the long-term effects of sustained ketosis on health, as well as considerations for nutrient diversity, need careful evaluation.

3. Balanced Diets for Overall Health: Emphasizing a balanced intake of macronutrients through a variety of whole foods contributes to overall health. Such diets provide essential nutrients, support metabolic function, and may reduce the risk of chronic diseases. The Mediterranean diet, characterized by a balanced ratio of carbohydrates, proteins, and fats from whole, nutrient-dense sources, exemplifies a dietary pattern linked to various health benefits.

Challenges and Solutions in Balancing Macronutrients:

While achieving a balanced intake of macronutrients is a fundamental aspect of nutrition, several challenges may arise, and proactive strategies are essential to address them:

1. Processed Foods and Nutrient Quality: Processed foods often lack the nutrient density of whole, unprocessed foods. Minimizing the consumption of heavily processed foods and focusing on whole, nutrient-dense options contribute to optimal macronutrient and micronutrient intake.

2. Hidden Macronutrients: Certain foods may contain hidden macronutrients, leading to unintended imbalances. Reading food labels, understanding the composition of meals, and being

mindful of ingredient choices help individuals make informed decisions and avoid unintended macronutrient excesses or deficiencies.

3. Individual Variation: Individual responses to macronutrient ratios and dietary patterns can vary. Monitoring how the body responds to different dietary approaches and making adjustments based on individual needs, preferences, and health goals is crucial.

4. Social and Cultural Influences: Social and cultural factors can influence dietary choices, making it challenging to maintain a balanced macronutrient profile. Open communication, education, and adapting traditional recipes to align with nutritional goals can help overcome these challenges.

Conclusion: Striking a Balance for a Healthier Tomorrow

Balancing macronutrients is not a rigid prescription but a dynamic and individualized approach to nutrition. It involves considering the unique needs of each person, understanding the interplay of macronutrients in health and disease, and making informed dietary choices that align with individual goals.

As we navigate the complexities of modern life, where dietary options are diverse and information is abundant, the importance of balancing macronutrients remains at the forefront of discussions on nutrition. Empowering individuals with the knowledge and tools to achieve a harmonious balance of nutrients supports their journey toward not just a life with more years but a life with more healthy and vibrant years.

In the quest for optimal health and well-being, let the guiding principles of balanced macronutrients be a compass, steering us toward a healthier and more fulfilling tomorrow—one plate at a time.

Ensuring Micronutrient Intake

Nutrition is a multifaceted domain that extends beyond the mere consumption of calories. While macronutrients—carbohydrates, proteins, and fats—provide the energy necessary for bodily functions, micronutrients play a pivotal role in maintaining health and preventing deficiencies. Micronutrients, encompassing vitamins and minerals, are essential for various physiological processes, including immune function, bone health, and enzyme activity. This essay explores the significance of ensuring micronutrient intake, the consequences of deficiencies and excesses, and practical strategies for achieving a well-balanced and micronutrient-rich diet.

Micronutrients are essential compounds required by the body in relatively small amounts to maintain optimal health. They include vitamins and minerals, each serving unique functions in various physiological processes.

1. Vitamins:

- Fat-Soluble Vitamins:

- Vitamin A: Essential for vision, immune function, and skin health. Found in liver, sweet potatoes, carrots, and dark leafy greens.

- Vitamin D: Crucial for bone health and calcium absorption. Synthesized in the skin upon exposure to sunlight and found in fatty fish, egg yolks, and fortified foods.

- Vitamin E: Acts as an antioxidant, protecting cells from damage. Present in nuts, seeds, vegetable oils, and spinach.

- Vitamin K: Necessary for blood clotting and bone health. Found in green leafy vegetables, broccoli, and soybeans.

- Water-Soluble Vitamins:

- Vitamin C: A powerful antioxidant that supports immune function, collagen synthesis, and iron absorption. Abundant in citrus fruits, strawberries, bell peppers, and broccoli.

- B-Complex Vitamins: Including B1 (thiamine), B2 (riboflavin), B3 (niacin), B5 (pantothenic acid), B6 (pyridoxine), B7 (biotin), B9 (folate), and B12 (cobalamin). These vitamins are involved in energy metabolism, DNA synthesis, and red blood cell formation. Found in a variety of foods, including whole grains, meat, dairy, and leafy greens.

2. Minerals:

- Major Minerals:

- Calcium: Critical for bone and teeth formation, muscle function, and blood clotting. Found in dairy products, fortified plant milks, leafy greens, and tofu.

- Magnesium: Essential for muscle and nerve function, energy production, and bone health. Found in nuts, seeds, whole grains, and leafy greens.

- Sodium, Potassium, and Chloride: Electrolytes crucial for fluid balance, nerve function, and muscle contraction. Found in various foods, with potassium abundant in fruits and vegetables.

- Trace Minerals:

- Iron: Essential for oxygen transport in the blood. Found in red meat, poultry, beans, and fortified cereals.

- Zinc: Important for immune function, wound healing, and DNA synthesis. Found in meat, dairy, nuts, and legumes.

- Copper: Involved in iron metabolism and the formation of connective tissues. Found in organ meats, seafood, nuts, and seeds.

- Selenium: Acts as an antioxidant and supports thyroid function. Found in seafood, Brazil nuts, and grains.

The Importance of Micronutrient Intake:

Micronutrients play a crucial role in maintaining health and preventing a range of conditions associated with deficiencies. Their functions extend beyond energy metabolism and structural support to regulating biochemical reactions and supporting the body's defense mechanisms. Understanding the importance of micronutrient intake involves recognizing their specific roles in promoting well-being:

1. Immune Function: Micronutrients such as vitamins C, D, and E, as well as minerals like zinc and selenium, play key roles in supporting immune function. Deficiencies in these micronutrients can compromise the body's ability to mount an effective immune response, increasing susceptibility to infections.

2. Bone Health: Calcium, vitamin D, magnesium, and vitamin K are essential for maintaining strong and healthy bones. Inadequate intake of these micronutrients can lead to conditions like osteoporosis and increased fracture risk.

3. Energy Metabolism: B-Complex vitamins, including B1, B2, B3, B5, B6, B7, and B12, are crucial for energy metabolism. They participate in the conversion of nutrients into energy and support the proper functioning of enzymes involved in metabolic pathways.

4. Blood Clotting: Vitamin K is vital for blood clotting, preventing excessive bleeding in case of injury. Deficiencies in vitamin K can lead to impaired clotting and increased bleeding tendencies.

5. Antioxidant Defense: Antioxidant vitamins, such as vitamin C and E, help protect cells from oxidative stress by neutralizing free radicals. Adequate intake of these micronutrients contributes to overall cellular health and may reduce the risk of chronic diseases.

Consequences of Micronutrient Deficiencies:

Micronutrient deficiencies can have far-reaching consequences on health, leading to a range of conditions with varying degrees of sseverit. Common micronutrient deficiencies and their consequences include:

1. Iron Deficiency:

   - Consequence: Anemia

   - Iron deficiency can lead to anemia, characterized by fatigue, weakness, and impaired cognitive function. In severe cases, it may result in pale skin, shortness of breath, and compromised immune function.

2. Vitamin D Deficiency:

   - Consequence: Rickets (in children) and Osteomalacia (in adults)

   - Inadequate vitamin D can lead to poor bone development in children (rickets) and soft, weak bones in adults (osteomalacia). Vitamin D deficiency is also associated with increased susceptibility to infections and autoimmune conditions.

3. Vitamin C Deficiency:

   - Consequence: Scurvy

   - A deficiency in vitamin C can lead to scurvy, characterized by fatigue, swollen and bleeding gums, joint pain, and anemia. Severe cases can result in cardiovascular complications.

4. Iodine Deficiency:

- Consequence: Goiter and Hypothyroidism

- Insufficient iodine can lead to the enlargement of the thyroid gland (goiter) and hypothyroidism, which can result in fatigue, weight gain, and impaired cognitive function.

5. Vitamin A Deficiency:

- Consequence: Night Blindness and Xerophthalmia

- Inadequate vitamin A can lead to night blindness and, in severe cases, xerophthalmia—an eye condition that can lead to blindness. Vitamin A is also crucial for immune function.

Balancing Micronutrient Intake: Practical Strategies

Ensuring adequate micronutrient intake requires a conscientious approach to dietary choices and an understanding of the nutritional content of various foods. Here are practical strategies to achieve a well-balanced and micronutrient-rich diet:

1. Eat a Variety of Whole Foods: Consuming a diverse array of whole foods provides a broad spectrum of micronutrients. Include a colorful assortment of fruits, vegetables, whole grains, lean proteins, and healthy fats in your diet to maximize nutrient diversity.

2. Prioritize Nutrient-Dense Foods: Choose foods that are rich in nutrients per calorie. Nutrient-dense options include leafy greens, berries, nuts, seeds, lean proteins, and whole grains. These foods provide essential vitamins and minerals without excessive calories.

3. Limit Processed Foods: Processed foods often lack the nutritional density of whole foods and may be deficient in certain micronutrients. Minimize the consumption of heavily processed foods and focus on fresh, whole, and minimally processed options.

4. Consider Cooking Methods: Certain cooking methods can impact the nutrient content of foods. Opt for cooking methods like steaming, roasting, and sautéing to preserve the nutritional value of vegetables and proteins. Avoid overcooking, as prolonged heat exposure can lead to nutrient loss.

5. Be Mindful of Micronutrient-Rich Foods: Identify foods that are particularly rich in specific micronutrients and incorporate them into your diet. For example, fatty fish is an excellent source of omega-3 fatty acids, while nuts and seeds provide a range of vitamins and minerals.

6. Supplementation When Necessary: In certain situations, supplementation may be necessary to address specific micronutrient needs. For example, individuals with vitamin D deficiencies may require supplements. However, it's essential to consult with a healthcare professional before initiating supplementation.

7. Consider Individual Needs: Individual requirements for micronutrients vary based on factors such as age, gender, activity level, and health conditions. Pregnant women, for instance, may have increased needs for certain micronutrients. Tailoring dietary choices to individual needs ensures personalized and effective micronutrient intake.

Micronutrients in Different Life Stages:

Micronutrient needs evolve throughout different life stages, emphasizing the importance of adjusting dietary choices to meet changing requirements.

1. Infants and Children:

   - Adequate intake of micronutrients is crucial for growth and development.

   - Breast milk or fortified infant formulas provide essential vitamins and minerals.

   - Introduction of nutrient-dense foods as complementary feeding is essential to meet increasing nutrient needs.

2. Adolescents:

   - Rapid growth during adolescence requires increased intake of key micronutrients, including calcium, iron, and vitamin D.

   - Encouraging the consumption of dairy products, lean proteins, and fruits and vegetables supports overall health and development.

3. Adults:

   - Maintaining a balanced diet is essential for overall well-being and disease prevention.

   - Adequate intake of micronutrients supports immune function, bone health, and energy metabolism.

   - Calcium and vitamin D become particularly important for bone health, especially in postmenopausal women.

4. Seniors:

- Aging is associated with changes in nutrient absorption and metabolism.

- Calcium and vitamin D remain crucial for bone health, while vitamin B12 supplementation may be necessary for some seniors.

- A diet rich in antioxidants supports cognitive health and mitigates oxidative stress associated with aging.

Challenges in Micronutrient Intake and Solutions:

Despite the importance of micronutrient intake, several challenges can hinder optimal nutrition. Identifying these challenges and implementing practical solutions is essential for overcoming barriers to achieving adequate micronutrient intake:

1. Limited Access to Nutrient-Dense Foods:

  - Solution:

   - Promote community gardens and farmers' markets to increase access to fresh produce.

   - Advocate for policies that support affordable and nutritious food options in underserved communities.

2. Dietary Restrictions:

  - Solution:

   - Work with healthcare professionals or registered dietitians to ensure that dietary restrictions, such as those in vegetarian or vegan diets, are addressed with appropriate substitutes and supplements if necessary.

   - Educate individuals on how to meet their micronutrient needs within the constraints of their dietary preferences.

3. Food Insecurity:

  - Solution:

   - Support and advocate for initiatives that address food insecurity at the community and policy levels.

   - Encourage local organizations to establish food banks and distribution programs to provide nutrient-dense foods to those in need.

4. Limited Nutrition Education:

  - Solution:

   - Implement comprehensive nutrition education programs in schools and communities.

   - Promote the importance of nutrition education for healthcare professionals to enhance their ability to provide evidence-based dietary guidance.

Conclusion: Empowering Health Through Micronutrients

Ensuring micronutrient intake is not merely a dietary recommendation; it is a fundamental aspect of promoting health, preventing deficiencies, and supporting optimal physiological function. The intricate dance of vitamins and minerals orchestrates a symphony of biochemical reactions within the body, influencing everything from immune response to cognitive function.

As we navigate the complexities of modern life, with its myriad food choices and nutritional information, cultivating awareness about micronutrient intake becomes an empowering journey. From the early stages of life, where growth and development are paramount, to the golden years, where maintaining health and vitality takes precedence, the role of micronutrients remains central.

Chapter Seven

Plant-Based Plate: Tips and Menus for a Nutrient-Rich Lifestyle

The shift towards plant-based eating has gained widespread recognition for its potential health benefits, environmental sustainability, and ethical considerations. A plant-based plate emphasizes whole, plant-derived foods, including fruits, vegetables, grains, legumes, nuts, and seeds, while minimizing or excluding animal products. This essay delves into the principles of creating a plant-based plate, offers practical tips for transitioning to a plant-based lifestyle, and provides diverse menus that showcase the delicious and nutrient-rich possibilities of plant-centric eating.

The Plant-Based Plate: A Nutrient-Packed Canvas

Building a plant-based plate involves thoughtfully incorporating a variety of nutrient-dense foods to ensure a well-rounded and satisfying meal. The components of a plant-based plate can be divided into several key categories:

1. Vegetables:

   - Dark Leafy Greens: Kale, spinach, Swiss chard, and collard greens are rich in vitamins, minerals, and antioxidants.

   - Colorful Vegetables: Bell peppers, tomatoes, carrots, and broccoli add vibrant colors and a spectrum of nutrients to the plate.

2. Fruits:

   - Berries: Strawberries, blueberries, raspberries, and blackberries provide antioxidants and natural sweetness.

   - Citrus Fruits: Oranges, grapefruits, and lemons contribute vitamin C and a refreshing taste.

3. Whole Grains:

   - Quinoa: A complete protein source with a nutty flavor and versatile uses.

   - Brown Rice: Fiber-rich and a staple in many plant-based cuisines.

   - Oats: High in soluble fiber, supporting heart health and digestion.

4. Legumes:

   - Lentils: A protein powerhouse that pairs well with various dishes.

   - Chickpeas: Versatile legumes used in salads, curries, and snacks.

   - Black Beans: Rich in fiber and a great addition to soups, stews, and burritos.

5. Nuts and Seeds:

   - Almonds: Packed with healthy fats, protein, and essential nutrients.

   - Chia Seeds: High in omega-3 fatty acids and fiber, excellent for puddings and smoothies.

- Flaxseeds: A good source of omega-3s and lignans, promoting heart health.

6. Plant-Based Proteins:

  - Tofu: A versatile soy-based protein that takes on the flavors of its surroundings.

  - Tempeh: Fermented soy product with a nutty taste and firm texture.

  - Seitan: A high-protein meat substitute made from gluten.

7. Healthy Fats:

  - Avocado: Rich in monounsaturated fats, vitamins, and minerals.

  - Olive Oil: A staple in Mediterranean cuisine, providing heart-healthy fats.

  - Walnuts: Omega-3 fatty acids and antioxidants make walnuts a nutritious snack.

8. Herbs and Spices:

  - Basil, Cilantro, Parsley: Add freshness and flavor to dishes.

  - Turmeric, Cumin, Paprika: Spices with anti-inflammatory properties and diverse tastes.

Practical Tips for Transitioning to a Plant-Based Lifestyle:

Transitioning to a plant-based lifestyle is a gradual process that involves exploring new foods, flavors, and cooking techniques. Here are practical tips to facilitate a smooth transition:

1.Educate Yourself:

  - Learn about Nutritional Needs: Understand the essential nutrients found in plant-based foods and how to ensure a well-balanced diet.

  - Explore Plant-Based Cooking Techniques: Familiarize yourself with techniques such as sautéing, roasting, and blending to enhance the flavors and textures of plant-based ingredients.

2. Start Gradually:

  -Meatless Mondays: Begin by designating one day a week for plant-based meals and gradually increase the frequency.

  - Explore New Ingredients: Introduce a variety of grains, legumes, and vegetables to diversify your plant-based repertoire.

3. Focus on Whole Foods:

- Minimize Processed Foods: While convenient, processed plant-based foods may lack the nutritional benefits of whole foods. Emphasize whole grains, fresh produce, and minimally processed alternatives.

4. Experiment with Flavors:

- Herbs and Spices: Explore a variety of herbs and spices to add depth and flavor to plant-based dishes.

- Citrus and Vinegar: Use citrus fruits and vinegar to enhance taste without relying on excessive salt or sugar.

5. Plan Balanced Meals:

- Include a Variety of Colors: A vibrant plate is often indicative of diverse nutrients. Aim for a colorful mix of fruits and vegetables.

- Incorporate Protein Sources: Include plant-based proteins like beans, lentils, tofu, and tempeh to meet protein requirements.

6. Find Plant-Based Alternatives:

- Dairy Alternatives: Explore plant-based milk, yogurt, and cheese options made from almonds, soy, oats, or coconut.

- Meat Substitutes: Try plant-based alternatives like veggie burgers, plant-based sausages, and meatless ground options.

7. Connect with the Plant-Based Community:

- Join Online Communities: Engage with online forums, social media groups, and blogs dedicated to plant-based living for support, inspiration, and recipe ideas.

- Attend Local Events: Participate in local plant-based events, farmers' markets, or cooking classes to connect with like-minded individuals.

8. Meal Prep and Batch Cooking:

- Plan Ahead: Prepare plant-based meals in advance to make healthy choices more accessible during busy times.

- Batch Cooking: Cook large quantities of grains, beans, and vegetables to use in various dishes throughout the week.

Plant-Based Menus: A Culinary Journey

Creating a diverse and satisfying plant-based menu involves exploring a spectrum of flavors, textures, and cuisines. Here are three sample plant-based menus that showcase the versatility and deliciousness of plant-centric eating:

Menu 1: Mediterranean Delights

Appetizer:

- Mediterranean Hummus Platter

  - Hummus served with cherry tomatoes, cucumber slices, kalamata olives, and whole-grain pita bread.

Main Course:

- Grilled Eggplant and Zucchini Ratatouille

  - Layers of grilled eggplant, zucchini, tomatoes, and bell peppers drizzled with olive oil and fresh herbs.

Side Dish:

- Quinoa Tabbouleh Salad

  - Quinoa mixed with diced tomatoes, cucumbers, parsley, mint, and a lemon-tahini dressing.

Dessert:

- Fresh Fruit Salad with Mint

  - A refreshing mix of seasonal fruits topped with chopped mint.

Menu 2: Asian Fusion Feast

Appetizer:

- Edamame and Avocado Spring Rolls

  - Rice paper rolls filled with edamame, sliced avocado, carrots, and mint, served with a soy-ginger dipping sauce.

Main Course:

- Vegan Pad Thai

  - Stir

-fried rice noodles with tofu, bean sprouts, peanuts, and a tangy tamarind sauce.

Side Dish:

- Stir-Fried Sesame Broccoli

  - Broccoli florets stir-fried with sesame oil, garlic, and soy sauce.

Dessert:

- Coconut Mango Sticky Rice

  - Sweet sticky rice topped with ripe mango slices and a coconut milk drizzle.

Menu 3: South American Fiesta

Appetizer:

- Guacamole and Salsa with Baked Tortilla Chips

  - Homemade guacamole and salsa served with whole-grain baked tortilla chips.

Main Course:

- Black Bean and Corn Stuffed Peppers

  - Bell peppers filled with a mixture of black beans, corn, tomatoes, and spices, baked to perfection.

Side Dish:

- Quinoa and Avocado Salad

  - Quinoa salad with diced avocado, black beans, cherry tomatoes, and a lime-cilantro dressing.

Dessert:

- Chia Seed Pudding with Mixed Berries

  - Chia seed pudding made with almond milk, topped with a medley of mixed berries.

Conclusion: Cultivating a Plant-Centric Lifestyle

The plant-based plate is not merely a collection of ingredients; it is a canvas of creativity, flavor, and nourishment. Embracing a plant-centric lifestyle involves more than just the foods on your plate; it encompasses a holistic approach to well-being, sustainability, and ethical choices.

As individuals embark on the journey of transitioning to a plant-based lifestyle, the principles of balance, variety, and mindful eating become guiding lights. Through education, experimentation, and a connection with the vibrant plant-based community, one can discover the joy and abundance that a plant-based plate has to offer.

In a world where dietary choices have far-reaching implications for personal health and the planet, the plant-based plate stands as a symbol of conscious living—a choice that nourishes not only the body but also the interconnected web of life we all share. So, let the plant-based plate be an invitation to explore, savor, and celebrate the diverse and delicious world of plant-centric eating.

Chapter Eight

The Connection Between Plant-Powered Diets and Sustainability

In recent years, the intersection of dietary choices and environmental sustainability has emerged as a critical topic of discussion. As the global population continues to grow and concerns about climate change escalate, the need for sustainable food practices has become more apparent than ever. Plant-powered diets, characterized by a predominant or exclusive reliance on plant-based foods, have garnered attention not only for their potential health benefits but also for their positive impact on the planet. This essay explores the intricate connection between plant-powered diets and sustainability, examining how our food choices can play a pivotal role in nourishing both the planet and our individual well-being.

The Environmental Footprint of Food Choices

The food we consume has far-reaching implications for the environment, influencing land use, water resources, greenhouse gas emissions, and biodiversity. Traditional Western diets, often high in animal products, contribute significantly to environmental degradation. Livestock farming, particularly beef production, is a major driver of deforestation, habitat destruction, and water pollution. Additionally, the intensive use of resources in animal agriculture contributes substantially to greenhouse gas emissions, exacerbating climate change.

1. Land Use:

 - Deforestation for Livestock Grazing: Large-scale livestock farming necessitates vast expanses of land for grazing. In regions like the Amazon rainforest, substantial deforestation occurs to create pastureland, leading to biodiversity loss and habitat destruction.

 - Crop Cultivation for Animal Feed: Growing crops for animal feed demands extensive agricultural land. Corn, soy, and other feed crops require significant water and energy inputs.

2. Water Resources:

 - Water Intensity of Animal Agriculture: Livestock farming, particularly the production of beef, is water-intensive. The cultivation of feed crops, watering animals, and processing meat all contribute to substantial water consumption.

 - Water Pollution: Runoff from animal farms, containing waste and chemicals, can pollute water sources, negatively impacting aquatic ecosystems and human communities downstream.

3. Greenhouse Gas Emissions:

- Methane from Ruminant Digestion: Ruminant animals, such as cattle, produce methane during digestion. Methane is a potent greenhouse gas with a considerably higher warming potential than carbon dioxide over the short term.

- Energy Intensity of Animal Agriculture: The production, processing, and transportation of animal products require significant energy inputs, contributing to greenhouse gas emissions.

4. Biodiversity Loss:

- Habitat Destruction: The expansion of agricultural land for livestock farming often leads to the destruction of natural habitats, threatening biodiversity.

- Overfishing: The fishing industry, while not exclusive to plant-powered diets, can contribute to overfishing and depletion of marine resources.

Plant-Powered Diets: A Sustainable Alternative

Plant-powered diets, which prioritize plant-derived foods such as fruits, vegetables, whole grains, legumes, nuts, and seeds while minimizing or eliminating animal products, offer a more sustainable alternative to traditional diets. Several key aspects illustrate the sustainability of plant-powered diets:

1. Reduced Environmental Footprint:

- Land Use Efficiency: Plant-based agriculture tends to be more land-efficient compared to raising livestock. A greater variety of crops can be cultivated on a given area, utilizing land more effectively.

- Lower Water Intensity: Plant-based foods generally have a lower water footprint compared to animal products. Fruits, vegetables, and grains require less water to produce, contributing to water conservation.

2. Lower Greenhouse Gas Emissions:

- Reduced Methane Production: Plant-based diets, devoid of ruminant animals, significantly reduce methane emissions associated with digestion. This helps mitigate the warming potential of greenhouse gases.

- Energy Efficiency: The production and processing of plant-based foods often require fewer energy inputs, leading to lower overall greenhouse gas emissions.

3. Preservation of Biodiversity:

- Reduced Habitat Destruction: Plant-based agriculture typically involves less extensive land use, helping to preserve natural habitats and biodiversity.

- Crop Diversity: The cultivation of diverse crops for plant-based diets supports agroecosystems that promote biodiversity and resilience against pests and diseases.

4. Water Conservation:

- Efficient Water Use: Plant-based diets generally have a lower water footprint per calorie compared to diets rich in animal products. This is particularly important in regions facing water scarcity.

5. Mitigation of Overfishing:

- Reduced Dependence on Seafood: While plant-powered diets do not eliminate fishing, they often reduce the overall demand for seafood, contributing to efforts to mitigate overfishing and preserve marine ecosystems.

Health Benefits of Plant-Powered Diets

In addition to their environmental advantages, plant-powered diets are associated with various health benefits. The inclusion of nutrient-dense plant foods provides essential vitamins, minerals, fiber, and antioxidants, contributing to overall well-being and reducing the risk of chronic diseases. The health benefits of plant-powered diets include:

1. Cardiovascular Health:

- Reduced Saturated Fat Intake: Plant-based diets tend to be lower in saturated fats, which can contribute to improved cardiovascular health.

- High Fiber Content: Whole plant foods, such as fruits, vegetables, and whole grains, are rich in dietary fiber, which supports heart health by lowering cholesterol levels.

2. Weight Management:

- Lower Caloric Density: Plant-based diets, when focused on whole, unprocessed foods, often have a lower caloric density. This can aid in weight management and reduce the risk of obesity-related conditions.

3. Type 2 Diabetes Prevention:

- Improved Insulin Sensitivity: Plant-based diets may enhance insulin sensitivity, reducing the risk of type 2 diabetes. The fiber content of plant foods plays a role in stabilizing blood sugar levels.

4. Cancer Prevention:

- Antioxidant Protection: Plant foods are rich in antioxidants, which help protect cells from oxidative stress and may contribute to cancer prevention.

- Phytochemicals: Plant compounds such as phytochemicals have been associated with anti-cancer properties.

5. Digestive Health:

- Increased Fiber Intake: The fiber in plant foods supports digestive health by promoting regular bowel movements and a healthy gut microbiome.

- Prebiotics: Some plant foods contain prebiotics, fostering the growth of beneficial gut bacteria.

6. Longevity and Overall Well-Being:

- Nutrient Density: Plant-powered diets provide a high level of nutrients per calorie, contributing to overall health and longevity.

- Reduced Risk of Chronic Diseases: The consumption of plant foods is associated with a lower risk of chronic diseases, including cardiovascular disease, hypertension, and certain cancers.

Barriers and Challenges to Plant-Powered Diets

While the benefits of plant-powered diets for both the environment and health are substantial, various barriers and challenges can hinder widespread adoption. Addressing these challenges is crucial for promoting sustainable dietary choices on a global scale:

1. Cultural and Social Influences:

- Culinary Traditions: Dietary habits are often deeply rooted in cultural traditions, making it challenging for individuals to shift away from familiar animal-based dishes.

- Social Norms: Social gatherings, celebrations, and shared meals may center around animal products, creating social challenges for those adopting plant-powered diets.

2. Perceived Lack of Accessibility:

- Affordability: The perception that plant-based diets are more expensive can be a barrier, especially in regions where plant-based alternatives may be costlier than conventional animal products.

- Availability: Limited access to fresh produce and plant-based alternatives in certain areas may hinder individuals from adopting plant-powered diets.

3. Nutritional Concerns:

- Protein and Nutrient Adequacy: Some individuals may be concerned about obtaining adequate protein and essential nutrients on plant-powered diets. Education on proper nutrition is crucial to address these concerns.

- Vitamin B12 and Omega-3 Fatty Acids: Plant-based diets may require attention to sources of vitamin B12 and omega-3 fatty acids, which are primarily found in animal products.

4. Lack of Culinary Skills and Knowledge:

- Cooking Competence: Individuals who lack confidence or skills in plant-based cooking may find it challenging to prepare diverse and satisfying meals.

- Recipe Familiarity: A lack of familiarity with plant-based recipes and cooking techniques may deter individuals from embracing a plant-powered lifestyle.

5. Marketing and Dietary Misinformation:

- Influence of Food Industry: The marketing and promotion of animal products, processed foods, and fast food can influence dietary choices, contributing to the persistence of less sustainable and less healthy diets.

- Misinformation: Conflicting information about nutrition and dietary choices may lead to confusion and misinformation, making it difficult for individuals to make informed decisions.

Overcoming Challenges: Strategies for Promoting Plant-Powered Diets

Addressing the barriers to plant-powered diets requires a multifaceted approach involving education, accessibility, policy changes, and cultural shifts. Here are strategies to promote and support the adoption of plant-powered diets:

1. Educational Initiatives:

- Nutritional Education: Implement comprehensive nutritional education programs in schools, communities, and healthcare settings. Empower individuals with knowledge about the health benefits of plant-powered diets and how to achieve nutritional adequacy.

- Cooking Classes: Offer community-based cooking classes focused on plant-based recipes, teaching essential culinary skills and making plant-powered eating more accessible.

2. Policy Changes:

- Subsidies for Plant-Based Foods: Implement policies that provide subsidies for the production and distribution of plant-based foods, making them more affordable and accessible.

- Nutrition Labeling: Enhance nutrition labeling to clearly indicate the environmental impact of food products, empowering consumers to make informed choices.

3. Culinary Innovation:

- Plant-Based Alternatives: Encourage and support the development of innovative plant-based alternatives to traditional animal products, making it easier for individuals to transition without compromising taste or convenience.

- Collaboration with Chefs: Collaborate with chefs and culinary experts to create appealing and flavorful plant-based dishes that cater to diverse tastes.

4. Promotion of Local and Sustainable Agriculture:

- Community Gardens: Support community gardens and local agriculture to increase access to fresh, locally grown produce.

- Farmers' Markets: Promote farmers' markets and initiatives that connect consumers with local, sustainable, and plant-powered food sources.

5. Social and Cultural Influences:

- Cultural Integration: Integrate plant-powered dietary options into culinary traditions and cultural practices, fostering acceptance and adaptation.

- Celebrity Endorsement: Leverage the influence of celebrities and public figures to promote plant-powered lifestyles and challenge cultural norms.

6. Accessible Plant-Based Alternatives:

- Affordable Plant-Based Options: Work towards making plant-based alternatives affordable and widely available, ensuring that cost is not a barrier to adopting a plant-powered diet.

- Fast Food Partnerships: Collaborate with fast-food chains to introduce and promote plant-based options on their menus.

7. Public Awareness Campaigns:

- Media Campaigns: Launch media campaigns that highlight the environmental and health benefits of plant-powered diets, dispelling myths and providing factual information.

- Social Media Influencers: Engage social media influencers to promote plant-powered living, sharing personal stories, recipes, and tips.

8. School and Workplace Initiatives:

- Plant-Based Options in Cafeterias: Introduce plant-powered menu options in schools, universities, and workplaces, exposing individuals to diverse and appealing plant-based meals.

- Workplace Wellness Programs: Implement workplace wellness programs that educate employees about the benefits of plant-powered diets and provide resources for adopting healthier eating habits.

Conclusion: Cultivating a Sustainable Future Through Plant-Powered Diets

The connection between plant-powered diets and sustainability is a powerful catalyst for positive change, both for the health of individuals and the well-being of the planet. As we stand at the crossroads of environmental challenges and global health crises, the adoption of plant-powered diets emerges as a practical and impactful solution.

Embracing a plant-powered lifestyle is not merely a dietary choice; it is a conscious commitment to nourishing the Earth and safeguarding the health of current and future generations. The journey towards sustainability through plant-powered diets involves collaboration among individuals, communities, businesses, and policymakers to create a food system that prioritizes environmental stewardship, ethical considerations, and human well-being.

In this era of interconnected challenges, the shift towards plant-powered diets represents a beacon of hope—a tangible and achievable step towards a more sustainable and resilient future. It is a journey that calls for collective effort, innovation, and a shared vision of a world where the food we eat aligns harmoniously with the health of our bodies and the vitality of the planet we call home. Through mindful choices and informed actions, we have the power to cultivate a sustainable future—one plant-powered meal at a time.

Chapter Nine
Protein Myths and Realities

Protein is a fundamental component of the human diet, playing a crucial role in various physiological processes and serving as a building block for tissues, enzymes, hormones, and more. As interest in health and nutrition continues to grow, so does the plethora of information — both accurate and misleading — surrounding protein consumption. This essay aims to navigate the complex landscape of protein myths and realities, debunking common misconceptions and providing evidence-based insights into the importance, sources, and optimal intake of this essential nutrient.

Myth 1: More Protein Equals More Muscle

One pervasive myth in the fitness and nutrition world is the notion that consuming excessive amounts of protein automatically translates to more muscle mass. While protein is indeed vital for muscle repair and growth, the relationship between protein intake and muscle synthesis is more nuanced than the simplistic "more is better" perspective.

Reality: Optimal Protein Intake for Muscle Growth

Muscle protein synthesis is a dynamic process influenced by factors such as the type of protein consumed, timing, and individual needs. Research suggests that there is an upper limit to the amount of protein the body can use for muscle protein synthesis per meal, beyond which the excess may not confer additional benefits. Instead of focusing solely on increasing protein intake, individuals aiming for muscle growth should prioritize a balanced approach that includes resistance training, sufficient overall caloric intake, and strategic protein distribution throughout the day.

Myth 2: Plant-Based Diets Lack Adequate Protein

A common misconception is that individuals following plant-based diets, such as vegetarians and vegans, struggle to meet their protein needs due to a perceived lack of protein sources from plant foods.

Reality: Plant-Based Protein Adequacy

Contrary to the myth, plant-based diets can provide ample protein when well-planned. Various plant foods, including legumes, grains, nuts, seeds, and soy products, offer a diverse range of amino acids, the building blocks of proteins. Combining different plant protein sources throughout the day ensures that individuals on plant-based diets receive a complete array of essential amino

acids. Additionally, plant-based diets often contribute to other health benefits, such as increased fiber, antioxidants, and micronutrient intake.

Myth 3: Protein Supplements are Necessary for Everyone

With the booming market for protein supplements, there is a prevalent belief that everyone, regardless of their dietary habits or fitness level, needs to supplement their protein intake for optimal health.

Reality: Whole Foods First, Supplements Second

While protein supplements can be convenient for individuals with specific needs, such as athletes or those with increased protein requirements, they are not a one-size-fits-all solution. Whole foods should always be prioritized as the primary source of nutrients. Most individuals, even those engaged in regular exercise, can meet their protein needs through a well-balanced diet that includes a variety of whole foods. Protein supplements should be viewed as a supplement to, not a replacement for, a nutrient-dense diet.

Myth 4: All Proteins are Created Equal

Not all proteins are alike, and the myth that all protein sources are equally beneficial for health and muscle development oversimplifies the complexity of protein quality.

Reality: Complete vs. Incomplete Proteins

Proteins are made up of amino acids, and they can be classified as complete or incomplete based on their amino acid profile. Complete proteins, found in animal products such as meat, fish, eggs, and dairy, contain all essential amino acids in sufficient amounts. Incomplete proteins, found in plant sources like beans, grains, and nuts, may lack one or more essential amino acids. However, by combining different plant sources, individuals can easily obtain a complete set of amino acids, debunking the myth that plant-based proteins are inferior.

Myth 5: High-Protein Diets Always Lead to Weight Loss

The idea that consuming a high-protein diet is a guaranteed path to weight loss is prevalent in many dieting trends and weight loss programs.

Reality: Balance is Key

While protein plays a crucial role in weight management due to its satiating effect and potential impact on metabolism, the myth that a high-protein diet is a magic bullet for weight loss oversimplifies the complex factors influencing body composition. Sustainable weight loss is achieved through a combination of factors, including a well-rounded diet, regular physical activity,

and a healthy lifestyle. Relying solely on protein intake without addressing other aspects of one's lifestyle may yield limited and temporary results.

Myth 6: Protein Causes Kidney Damage

A longstanding myth is that high-protein diets can lead to kidney damage or worsen existing kidney conditions.

Reality: Protein and Kidney Health

Research has shown that individuals with normal kidney function can safely consume high-protein diets without adverse effects on kidney health. However, for those with pre-existing kidney conditions, moderation in protein intake may be advised. It's essential to consider individual health status, consult healthcare professionals, and monitor kidney function regularly when making significant changes to protein intake. In the absence of kidney issues, protein consumption within recommended limits is unlikely to cause harm.

Myth 7: All Protein Needs to Come from Animal Sources

A pervasive belief is that animal products are the superior and necessary source of protein, and plant-based proteins are inferior.

Reality: Diverse Protein Sources

A diverse array of protein sources, including both animal and plant-based options, can contribute to a well-balanced and nutritious diet. While animal products provide complete proteins with all essential amino acids, plant-based proteins offer additional benefits such as fiber, antioxidants, and lower saturated fat content. A diet that combines both plant and animal proteins can meet nutritional needs while promoting overall health and sustainability.

Myth 8: You Need Protein Right After a Workout

The post-workout "anabolic window" myth suggests that protein must be consumed immediately after exercise to maximize muscle protein synthesis and recovery.

Reality: Nutrient Timing is Secondary

While nutrient timing can play a role in certain contexts, the overall daily distribution of protein intake is more important than immediate post-exercise consumption. The body's ability to utilize protein for muscle repair and growth extends beyond the narrow post-workout window. As long as individuals meet their daily protein requirements through a well-rounded diet, the exact timing of protein consumption becomes a secondary consideration.

Myth 9: Protein Causes Osteoporosis

There is a misconception that high protein intake contributes to bone loss and the development of osteoporosis.

Reality: Protein and Bone Health

Research indicates that protein is crucial for maintaining bone health, and moderate protein intake does not have negative effects on bone density. In fact, adequate protein intake is associated with improved bone mineral density and a reduced risk of fractures. However, it's essential to balance protein intake with other nutrients, including calcium and vitamin D, to support overall bone health.

Myth 10: Children Need Less Protein than Adults

The myth that children require less protein than adults is a misconception that can impact the nutritional needs of growing individuals.

Reality: Protein Needs During Growth

Children and adolescents undergo rapid growth and development, necessitating adequate protein intake to support muscle, bone, and tissue formation. In some cases, children may require more protein per unit of body weight than adults. Providing protein-rich foods as part of a balanced diet is essential for meeting the nutritional needs of growing individuals and ensuring proper development.

Conclusion

Protein myths are pervasive in the realm of nutrition, often fueled by misinformation, fad diets, and oversimplifications. Navigating the complex landscape of protein requires a nuanced understanding of individual needs, diverse protein sources, and the broader context of overall dietary patterns. By dispelling common myths and embracing evidence-based realities, individuals can make informed choices about their protein intake, promoting both their health and well-being. As nutritional science continues to evolve, staying informed and critically evaluating dietary advice is paramount for making decisions that align with individual goals and contribute to long-term health.

Overcoming Nutritional Challenges

Nutrition is a cornerstone of overall health and well-being, influencing every aspect of our lives from physical vitality to mental clarity. However, the journey to optimal nutrition is riddled with challenges, both individual and systemic. This essay delves into the multifaceted realm of overcoming nutritional challenges, addressing issues ranging from food accessibility and affordability to the prevalence of misinformation and lifestyle factors that impact dietary choices. By understanding and proactively addressing these challenges, individuals and communities can pave the way towards a healthier and more nourished future.

1. Food Accessibility and Affordability

Challenge: Food Deserts and Limited Access

In various regions globally, individuals face the challenge of living in food deserts—areas with limited access to affordable, nutritious food. The lack of grocery stores, farmers' markets, and fresh produce options in these areas contributes to a reliance on convenience stores and fast food outlets, often leading to poor dietary choices.

Overcoming the Challenge: Community Initiatives and Policy Changes

Community-driven initiatives play a crucial role in addressing food accessibility challenges. Establishing community gardens, farmers' markets, and local co-ops can increase access to fresh, locally sourced produce. Additionally, advocating for policy changes that incentivize grocery stores to operate in underserved areas helps create a more equitable food landscape.

2. Nutrition Education and Misinformation

Challenge: Conflicting Nutritional Information

In the era of information overload, individuals are bombarded with conflicting advice on nutrition. Misinformation, often fueled by fad diets and pseudoscientific claims, contributes to confusion about healthy dietary choices.

Overcoming the Challenge: Science-Based Education and Media Literacy

Promoting nutrition education grounded in scientific evidence is essential to overcome misinformation. Integrating nutrition education into school curricula and workplace wellness programs can empower individuals to make informed choices. Moreover, fostering media literacy skills helps individuals critically evaluate nutritional information, distinguishing between evidence-based recommendations and marketing-driven myths.

3. Cultural and Social Influences

Challenge: Cultural Norms and Social Pressures

Cultural norms and social pressures heavily influence dietary choices, creating challenges for individuals attempting to adopt healthier eating habits. Traditional diets often rooted in cultural practices may clash with modern nutritional recommendations.

Overcoming the Challenge: Cultural Integration and Social Support

Efforts to integrate nutritional education with cultural practices can bridge the gap between tradition and optimal nutrition. Additionally, building social support networks that encourage healthier eating habits can empower individuals to navigate cultural and social influences successfully.

4. Busy Lifestyles and Convenience Foods

Challenge: Time Constraints and Convenience-Centric Diets

Modern lifestyles characterized by hectic schedules often lead individuals to prioritize convenience over nutrition. Fast food, processed snacks, and pre-packaged meals become go-to options, contributing to suboptimal dietary patterns.

Overcoming the Challenge: Meal Planning and Culinary Skills Education

Empowering individuals with meal planning skills and culinary education fosters a shift towards healthier, home-cooked meals. Educational programs that teach efficient cooking techniques and emphasize the importance of balanced, nutritious meals enable individuals to make healthier choices despite time constraints.

5. Environmental and Sustainability Concerns

Challenge: Environmental Impact of Food Choices

The environmental impact of food production, including issues like deforestation, water usage, and greenhouse gas emissions, poses a significant challenge. Diets high in animal products, particularly red meat, contribute to environmental degradation.

Overcoming the Challenge: Plant-Powered Diets and Sustainable Practices

Encouraging the adoption of plant-powered diets, which have a lower environmental footprint, is a key strategy. Promoting sustainable agricultural practices, reducing food waste, and supporting local, eco-friendly food systems contribute to a more environmentally conscious approach to nutrition.

6. Dietary Restrictions and Allergies

Challenge: Dietary Restrictions and Food Allergies

Individuals with dietary restrictions, whether due to health conditions or personal choices, face challenges in finding suitable and enjoyable food options. Food allergies add an additional layer of complexity, requiring careful attention to ingredient lists and food preparation methods.

Overcoming the Challenge: Diverse and Inclusive Food Options

Creating a diverse and inclusive food landscape that caters to various dietary preferences and restrictions is crucial. Restaurants, food manufacturers, and culinary professionals can play a role by offering a variety of options that accommodate different dietary needs without compromising flavor or nutritional value.

7. Economic Disparities and Nutritional Inequality

Challenge: Economic Barriers to Healthy Eating

Economic disparities contribute to nutritional inequality, with individuals facing financial constraints often resorting to lower-cost, energy-dense but nutrient-poor food options. The high cost of fresh produce and healthier alternatives exacerbates this challenge.

Overcoming the Challenge: Economic Policies and Community Programs

Implementing economic policies that make nutritious foods more affordable, such as subsidies for fresh produce, can help alleviate this challenge. Community programs, including food banks and initiatives providing affordable, healthy meal options, contribute to addressing nutritional inequality at the grassroots level.

8. Emotional and Psychological Factors

Challenge: Emotional Eating and Psychological Barriers

Emotional and psychological factors, such as stress, anxiety, and emotional eating, play a significant role in dietary choices. These factors can lead to the consumption of comfort foods high in sugars and fats, negatively impacting overall health.

Overcoming the Challenge: Mental Health Support and Mindful Eating Practices

Integrating mental health support into overall wellness programs is crucial. Mindful eating practices, including awareness of emotional triggers and cultivating a healthy relationship with food, help individuals overcome psychological barriers to healthy eating.

Conclusion: A Holistic Approach to Optimal Nutrition

Overcoming nutritional challenges requires a holistic and multifaceted approach that addresses individual behaviors, societal norms, economic disparities, and environmental considerations. By fostering a culture of nutrition education, promoting sustainable practices, and advocating for policies that prioritize food accessibility and affordability, we can collectively navigate the path to optimal health. Empowering individuals to make informed, mindful, and nourishing choices contributes not only to personal well-being but also to the creation of a healthier, more equitable global food landscape.

www.ingramcontent.com/pod-product-compliance
Lightning Source LLC
Chambersburg PA
CBHW061000260726

48661CB00005B/1963